O A P L
OXFORD AMERICAN PSYCHIATRY LIBRARY

ADHD

O A P L

OXFORD AMERICAN PSYCHIATRY LIBRARY

ADHD

James J. McGough, M.D., M.S.

Professor of Clinical Psychiatry and Biobehavioral Sciences
David Geffen School of Medicine and
Semel Institute for Neuroscience and Human Behavior at UCLA

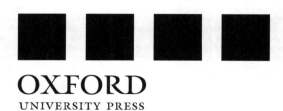

OXFORD
UNIVERSITY PRESS

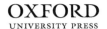

Oxford University Press is a department of the University of
Oxford. It furthers the University's objective of excellence in research,
scholarship, and education by publishing worldwide.

Oxford   New York
Auckland   Cape Town   Dar es Salaam   Hong Kong   Karachi
Kuala Lumpur   Madrid   Melbourne   Mexico City   Nairobi
New Delhi   Shanghai   Taipei   Toronto

With offices in
Argentina   Austria   Brazil   Chile   Czech Republic   France   Greece
Guatemala   Hungary   Italy   Japan   Poland   Portugal   Singapore
South Korea   Switzerland   Thailand   Turkey   Ukraine   Vietnam

Oxford is a registered trademark of Oxford University Press
in the UK and certain other countries.

Published in the United States of America by
Oxford University Press
198 Madison Avenue, New York, NY 10016

Library of Congress Cataloging-in-Publication Data
McGough, James J., author.
ADHD / James J. McGough.
   p. ; cm.—(Oxford American psychiatry library)
Attention deficit hyperactivity disorder
Includes bibliographical references.
ISBN 978–0–19–996990–6 (alk. paper)
I. Title.   II. Title: Attention deficit hyperactivity disorder.   III. Series: Oxford American
psychiatry library. [DNLM: 1.   Attention Deficit Disorder with Hyperactivity. WS 350.8.A8]
RC394.A85
616.85'89—dc23
2014006486

For Caitlin and Daniel

Contents

Acknowledgments

I wish to express appreciation to my students and colleagues, Drs. Peter Chung, Carl Fleisher, Roya Ijadi-Maghsoodi, Jessica Jeffrey, Sandra Loo, Smitta Patel, Gregory Sayer, Benjamin Schneider, Thomas Spencer, Mark Stein, and Timothy Wilens, who helped guide my writing and provided comments on earlier versions of this manuscript.

J.M.

Disclosure

The author has served on advisory boards or as a consultant to Akili Interactive, Merck & Co., Neurovance, Shionogi & Co., Sunovion Pharmaceuticals, Targacept, and Theravance, and has received research support from NeuroSigma Inc., Purdue Pharma, Shionogi Pharmaceuticals, Supurnus Pharmaceuticals, and Shire Pharmaceuticals.

Any discussion of off-label medication use contained herein is identified as such.

O A P L

OXFORD AMERICAN PSYCHIATRY LIBRARY

ADHD

Chapter 1

Introduction

Key Points

- Attention-deficit/hyperactivity disorder (ADHD) is a well-validated and commonly occurring brain-based disorder with significant life consequences.
- The scientific basis supporting our understanding and management of ADHD is of the strongest demonstrated among mental and behavioral disorders.

Attention-deficit/hyperactivity disorder (ADHD) is a frequently occurring, brain-based, neurodevelopmental disorder with substantial negative consequences for individual and public health. Once viewed as a childhood condition, it is now recognized that a majority of cases persist throughout adolescence and adulthood. The lifelong impact of ADHD often extends beyond the disorder's defining features of developmentally inappropriate levels of inattention and/or hyperactivity and impulsivity. Having ADHD is associated with significant added risk for developing other mental health disorders, as well as functional impairments, across a range of life domains. These include educational attainment, social skills, occupational success, personal relationships, parenting, personal safety, and general health. Societal economic burdens associated with ADHD are considerable. The National Institute of Mental Health (NIMH) has described ADHD as a major public health concern.[1]

The high community prevalence of ADHD suggests that there are affected patients in virtually every clinical practice in every medical specialty. Nonetheless, comprehensive education about ADHD is largely limited to specialized programs in child and adolescent psychiatry and behavioral pediatrics. Other clinicians, notably some in general pediatrics and other primary care disciplines, gain ADHD expertise through self-initiated learning and patient-driven experience. The standard in most general psychiatry and pediatric residency programs is to cover the topic with a limited number of lectures, with few opportunities for comprehensive and continuous clinical experience.

Misinformation about ADHD abounds. Some assert that ADHD is not real. Critics variably maintain that childhood inattention and hyperactivity are normal, the diagnosis is subjective, behaviors attributed to ADHD arise when parents and teachers fail to maintain appropriate discipline, older students fake symptoms to obtain academic advantages or performance-enhancing drugs, adults are similarly drug seeking or looking to excuse various life failures, or that the condition represents a conspiracy by pharmaceutical companies and organized psychiatry to increase medication sales.

ADHD, in fact, is among the most scientifically validated psychiatric disorders.[2] Its diagnostic reliability is well demonstrated and on par with many conditions in general medicine. The biological underpinnings of ADHD are as well demonstrated, or better demonstrated, as any other psychiatric disorder. Similarly, the accumulated evidence base for its clinical management is of the strongest in mental health. Medications for ADHD have been used for over 70 years in millions of patients annually, creating an indisputable record of real-world safety and positive benefit. There are more double-blind, placebo-controlled medication studies in ADHD than for any other childhood condition. Treatment effect sizes are double those typically seen with more widely prescribed medications for depression and schizophrenia.

The development of clinical acumen for management of any medical condition is best achieved with supervised experience and long-term contact with large numbers of patients. These cannot be replaced by any book or series of lectures. This text is an introduction to the basic and clinical sciences of ADHD. It is organized to inform on phenomenology, neurobiology, assessment, and approaches to treatment that provide the necessary background for optimal patient management. While primarily intended for students, trainees, and early-career clinicians, relevant information is succinctly summarized in key points, boxes, tables, and figures for the benefit of the inexperienced and experienced alike. Key references and suggestions for further reading are provided for those seeking additional information or greater understanding of presented topics.

References

1. Diagnosis and treatment of attention deficit hyperactivity disorder. *NIH Consensus Statement*. 1998;16:1–37.
2. Goldman LS, Genel M, Bezman RJ, Slanetz PJ. Diagnosis and treatment of attention-deficit/hyperactivity disorder in children and adolescents. Council on Scientific Affairs, American Medical Association. *JAMA*. 1998;279:1100–1107.

Chapter 2

Historical Perspectives

Key Points

- Clinical descriptions consistent with ADHD have existed for over 200 years.
- Terms used to describe what we recognize as ADHD evolved in response to emerging science and changing conceptions about mental and behavioral disorders.
- For most of its history, ADHD has been recognized as largely brain based and biologically driven.

Descriptions of behaviors that we would now recognize as ADHD have existed for at least 200 years (Fig. 2.1). The names given to this syndrome have changed, generally in response to evolving conceptions about etiology and phenomenology but also in response to shifting cultural and political approaches to understanding emotional and behavioral disorders (Table 2.1). One consistent theme throughout most of this history is the view that ADHD is a biologically driven, brain-based disorder.

Pre-20th-Century Descriptions

The earliest known clinical description of what is now understood as ADHD might be found in an 18th-century medical text authored by the German physician Melchior Adam Weikard.[1] Published no later than 1775, Weikard's textbook *Der Philosophische Arzt* broke with prevailing opinion in suggesting that disorders of emotion and behavior arose from medical and physiological causes, not from astrological influences of the moon, stars, and planets. In his chapter on attention problems, Weikard characterized patients with attention deficits as "unwary, careless, and flighty." Additionally, these patients were jumpy, impulsive, highly distractible, and deficient in completing tasks. Much of this anticipates ADHD symptoms described in the *Diagnostic and Statistical Manual of Mental Disorders*, fourth edition (*DSM-IV*). Weikard speculated that these behaviors were due to either dysregulation of cerebral fibers resulting from overstimulation or a general lack of discipline early in childhood. He further observed that attention problems appeared to decrease with age.

A second 18th-century reference published in 1795 by the Scottish physician Sir Alexander Crichton described a syndrome characterized by abnormal degrees of inattention and distractibility.[2] These problems began early in life, interfered with education, diminished with age, and were believed to result

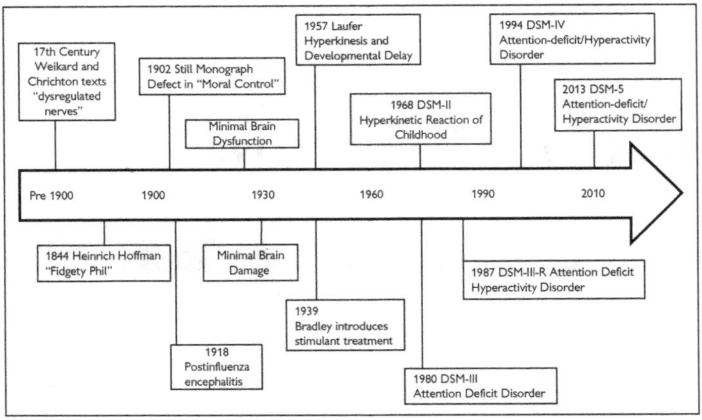

Figure 2.1 ADHD timeline.

Table 2.1 Changing Terms That Describe ADHD

Time Period	Classification	Term	Defining Features
1920s–1930s		Minimal brain damage	Behavior caused by structural brain lesions
1930s–1940s		Minimal brain dysfunction	Behavior caused by functional brain impairment
1950s		Hyperkinesis/ hyperkinetic syndrome	Brain-based developmental delay usually outgrown by adolescence
1960s	DSM-II	Hyperkinetic reaction of childhood	Behavioral reaction to unsupportive environments
1980s	DSM-III	Attention-deficit disorder (ADD)	Symptoms of inattention, impulsivity, hyperactivity. Could be diagnosed with (ADD/H) or without (ADD/WO) hyperactivity
	DSM-III-R	Attention-deficit/ hyperactivity disorder (ADHD)	Minimum number of combined inattentive, impulsive, hyperactive symptoms
1990s	DSM-IV	Attention-deficit/ hyperactivity disorder (ADHD)	Predominately inattentive, hyperactive/impulsive, and combined subtypes
2010s	DSM-5	Attention-deficit/ hyperactivity disorder (ADHD)	Criteria more developmentally sensitive for older patients.

from dysregulated "sensibility of the nerves." Associated difficulties included unusual levels of impulsivity, restlessness, and emotional reactivity.

In 1844 the German pediatrician Heinrich Hoffman published an illustrated storybook for children titled *Struwelpeter*, which contained a series of stories and pictures originally created to amuse crying children during physical examinations. One of these, "Fidgety Phil," depicted disruption at a family's dinner due to a boy's restlessness and lack of attention. The parent's angry response to their son's disruptions reflects family conflicts typically seen with an ADHD-affected child. "Fidgety Phil" suggests that observant clinicians have long recognized ADHD-like behaviors and related effects.[2]

Early 20th Century: Defects of Moral Control, Postencephalitic Behavior, and Minimal Brain Disorder

The first modern medical description of what is probably ADHD is attributed to the physician Sir George Frederick Still, regarded as the father of British pediatrics. In a series of lectures in 1902, Still discussed emotional and behavioral disorders of childhood in terms of "an abnormal defect of moral control" thought to reflect some level of physical brain damage.[3] Still viewed "moral control" as an intellectual capacity that restrained an individual's actions in the service of overall societal well-being. He described a group of children whose difficulties with inattention and impulsivity occurred without any specific intellectual or physical impairment. These children exhibited additional behaviors commonly associated with ADHD, including emotional reactivity and rage attacks, low frustration tolerance, and aggression. While some of these features are also consistent with oppositional defiant disorder, conduct disorder, or antisocial personality, the general consensus is that some cases had clear ADHD. Still's most significant contributions to our historical understanding of ADHD were his emphasis on a child-specific category of mental illness and the attribution of these behavioral difficulties to brain-based dysfunction.

Other early 20th-century events further contributed to an emerging view that problems with inattention and impulse control resulted from physical brain damage.[2] The first was an observed correlation between perinatal events, such as anoxia or birth defects, and subsequent behavioral and learning difficulties. Secondly, problems with inattention, distractibility, and mood lability were seen in soldiers who sustained head injuries during World War I, further illustrating the perceived link between brain injury and abnormal behavior. Additional evidence was seen in children who survived the flu pandemic of 1918 and subsequently developed a postencephalitic behavioral syndrome typified by inattention, poor motor control, moodiness, and restlessness. Building on Still's earlier work, these and other events contributed to an emerging view in the 1930s and 1940s that deviant behavior resulted from subtle damage to the brain. Children with long-standing and pervasive problems with attention and behavior were increasingly seen as suffering from minimal brain damage.

Although early 20th-century scientific investigations failed to identify specific areas of brain damage that led to inattention and overactivity, one research effort led to the serendipitous discovery of the positive effects of stimulant medications on hyperactive children. In the late 1930s, Dr. Charles Bradley, medical director of the Emma Pendleton Bradley Home in East Providence, Rhode Island, identified a group of youth with "emotional problems" and other learning and behavioral difficulties that were not explained by distinct neurological disorders. In investigating these children, Bradley obtained pneumoencephalograms to assess possible structural brain lesions. Bradley believed he could possibly reduce development of postprocedure headaches with amphetamine (Benzedrine®) administration, which he felt might stimulate the choroid plexus to replace lost cerebrospinal fluid. Amphetamine had a negligible impact on headaches, but teachers in the hospital's school observed striking behavioral improvements in some children. Bradley subsequently initiated a prospective trial, and in 1937 he reported significant behavioral and academic improvements in a majority of the children given amphetamine treatment.[4] One unfortunate consequence of this discovery was development of the mistaken belief that stimulants led to "paradoxical calming" in hyperactive children. This idea was later proven false when research showed that stimulants improved attention and motor restlessness in almost everyone. Bradley's discovery ultimately led to introduction in the 1950s and 1960s of other ADHD stimulants, including methamphetamine (Desoxyn®), dextroamphetamine (Dexedrine®), and the nonamphetamine methylphenidate (Ritalin®).

1950s: Minimal Brain Dysfunction, Hyperkinesis, and Developmental Delay

Emerging investigations in the 1950s questioned whether all children with abnormal behavior had underlying brain damage, even in the absence of demonstrated neurological lesions. New views suggested that functional as opposed to structural brain deficits caused behavioral difficulties, leading to a redefinition of "minimal brain damage" as "minimal brain dysfunction (MBD)."[2] The concept of MBD also proved unsatisfactory, as the category was too heterogeneous and likely to subsume a range of various behavioral, learning, and language disorders. In 1957, Laufer and Denhoff proposed that hyperactivity was the defining characteristic of the syndrome and introduced terms such as "hyperkinetic impulse disorder," "hyperkinesis," or a "hyperkinetic syndrome."[5] While still viewed as resulting from underlying brain pathology, the hyperkinetic syndrome was conceptualized as a developmental delay generally outgrown by adolescence. This remained the prevailing view well into the 1990s when evidence on the adult persistence of ADHD gained wide acceptance.

1960s–1970s: *DSM-II* Hyperkinetic Reaction of Childhood

The original *DSM* was published in 1952 to provide a common nomenclature for psychiatric illness. The manual contained only one childhood diagnosis, "adjustment reaction of childhood/adolescence." A second edition (*DSM-II*), published in 1968, described a categorical grouping "behavior disorders of childhood-adolescence," which included the diagnosis "hyperkinetic reaction of childhood." This disorder was characterized by a short attention span, restlessness, and hyperactivity. The clear implication was that these behaviors arose in reaction to unsupportive social environments, particularly caused by inadequate parenting or other parental conflict. This idea was consistent with prevailing views of the time that attributed most psychopathology to early developmental and social causes. This is the only period when ADHD behaviors were ascribed more to environmental and social causes rather than biological ones.

1980s: *DSM-III* Attention-Deficit Disorder and *DSM-III-R* Attention-Deficit/Hyperactivity Disorder

The third edition of the *DSM* (*DSM-III*) was the first classification system developed on broad-based scientific evidence. A major goal of *DSM-III* was to improve the reliability of psychiatric diagnoses, with an expectation that this would enhance research and standardize approaches to treatment. Expert panels in each diagnostic area proposed criteria that defined the various conditions. Some experts in childhood psychopathology noted that problems with attention sometimes occurred independently from hyperactive and impulsive symptoms, and they argued that the disorder is more a problem of inattention than hyperactivity. The previously named "hyperkinetic reaction" was redefined as attention-deficit disorder (ADD). Two subtypes were defined, that is, either with hyperactivity (ADD/H) or without it (ADD/WO). *DSM-III* proposed separate symptom lists for problems with inattention, impulsivity, and hyperactivity, and required some symptoms from each group for a diagnosis of ADD/H or from inattention and impulsivity only for those diagnosed with ADD/WO. In the 1987 revision of *DSM-III* (*DSM-III-R*), these symptoms were combined into a single set and diagnosis was determined by meeting a minimum number of total symptoms. *DSM-III-R* also reemphasized problems with hyperactivity and renamed the condition attention-deficit/hyperactivity disorder (ADHD). The name ADHD continues today as the official designation of this syndrome, but it is the cause of endless confusion when individuals lack hyperactive or impulsive symptoms.

1990s: *DSM-IV* Attention-Deficit/Hyperactivity Disorder

The fourth edition of the DSM (*DSM-IV*) was based in part on clinical field trials of proposed diagnostic criteria that demonstrated that ADHD symptoms appeared to separate into two domains, that is, inattentive and hyperactive/impulsive. This led to creation of the predominately inattentive, predominately hyperactive/impulsive, and combined ADHD subtypes. The minimal number of symptoms required for diagnosis was set at the 93rd percentile of symptom counts among school-aged children, which approximated two standard deviations above the mean for that group. Other *DSM-IV* criteria established that ADHD symptoms and related impairments must have been present by age 7, were evident in multiple settings, and were not better explained by other psychiatric disorders.

DSM-IV ADHD criteria provided a basis for significant advances in phenomenological and neurobiological research (see Chapter 4). Numerous investigations based on *DSM-IV* demonstrated that the disorder is largely heritable with clear genetic underpinnings. Both structural and functional imaging studies repeatedly revealed consistent differences between groups with and without the disorder. Longitudinal and phenomenological studies increasingly demonstrated that in a majority of cases ADHD persists into adulthood.

21st Century: *DSM-5*

The fifth edition of the *DSM* (*DSM-5*) made slight revisions to existing diagnostic criteria, primarily in response to an abundance of scientific findings (see Chapter 5). The syndrome name remained unchanged. Symptom descriptions were similarly unchanged, although clarifications were made to capture developmental changes with increasing age. The age of onset criterion was modified to require recognition of some symptoms prior to age 12, instead of the age 7 requirement for onset of symptoms and impairment described in *DSM-IV*. The number of symptoms necessary for diagnosis was reduced for older individuals to improve the criteria's developmental sensitivity. There was clear recognition that ADHD frequently occurs in adults, and descriptions of associated impairments were expanded to reflect more accurately the problems and concerns of older patients. Slight modifications were made to subtype definitions in favor of current symptom presentations. While the biological basis of ADHD was increasingly appreciated, diagnosis of the disorder remained dependent on careful assessment of clinical symptoms.

References

1. Barkley RA, Peters H. The earliest reference to ADHD in the medical literature? Melchior Adam Weikard's description in 1775 of "attention deficit" (Mangel der Aufmerksamkeit, Attentio Volubilis). *J Atten Disord*. 2012;16:623–630.

2. Lang KW, Reichl S, Lange KM, Tucha L, Tucha O. The history of attention deficit hyperactivity disorder. *Atten Defic Hyperact Disord*. 2010;2:241–255.

3. Still GF. Some abnormal psychical conditions in children: the Goulstonian lectures. *Lancet*. 1902;1:1008–1012.

4. Bradley C. The behavior of children receiving benzedrine. *Am J Psychiatry*. 1937;94:577–585.

5. Laufer MW, Denhoff E. Hyperkinetic behavior syndrome in children. *J Pediatr*. 1957;50:463–474.

Chapter 3

Epidemiology and Burden

Key Points

- Worldwide prevalence estimates for ADHD range from 3% to 10% for school-age children and 4% to 5% for adults.
- ADHD is associated with increased lifetime risk for anxiety, depression, substance abuse, and impulse control disorders.
- Individuals with ADHD suffer greater numbers of accidents and other medical difficulties, and they also exhibit higher levels of risky behavior, particularly with driving and sexual activity.
- ADHD creates substantial economic costs for affected individuals, families, and society.

ADHD is the most common behavioral disorder of childhood and in the majority of cases persists into adolescence and adulthood. Across the life span, ADHD is associated significant comorbidity, functional impairments, and increased economic burden. Key demographic facts for ADHD are summarized in Box 3.1.

Prevalence

The estimated prevalence of ADHD among school-age children ranges from 3% to 10%, with a 5.3% estimated worldwide mean.[1] Variability among estimates is due in part to differences in approaches to data collection, which include structured diagnostic interviews, parent or teacher rating scales, or parent histories that their child has received a clinician's diagnosis. One study from the US Centers for Disease Control and based on parent reports found that 9.5% of children and adolescents between ages 4 and 17 years had been given clinical diagnoses of ADHD.[2]

The prevalence of ADHD is higher in boys than in girls, with ratios of 9 to 1 and 3 to 1 in clinic and community samples, respectively. Boys might be overrepresented in clinics because they more frequently exhibit hyperactive/impulsive symptoms that create overt difficulties in school and with peers. Girls with fewer hyperactive/impulsive symptoms might have equal or greater impairments from inattention, but they are less likely to disturb parents and teachers and be referred for clinical evaluation. Boys are almost three times as likely as girls to receive a prescription.

ADHD occurs in all racial, ethnic, and socioeconomic groups and is not a function of intellectual ability.[2] Reported rates are somewhat higher in poorer

Box 3.1 ADHD: Key Demographics		
Prevalence estimates	School-age children	3%–10%
	Adults	2%–7%
Male/female ratios	School-age clinic samples	9:1
	School-age community samples	3:1
	Adult clinic samples	1:1
	Adult community samples	3:2
2007 estimate of affected youth ages 4–17 years		5.4 million (9.5%)
2007 estimate of youth ages 4–17 years on ADHD medication		2.2 million
2010 estimate of total cost of ADHD to US economy		$143–$266 billion

families and those headed by single mothers. Hispanic families are less likely to report that a child has been diagnosed, although it is unclear whether this reflects lower ADHD prevalence or cultural bias against evaluation and treatment.

ADHD symptoms often decrease as affected individuals enter adolescence. Point prevalence estimates suggest that rates of ADHD are lower in adolescents than in prepubertal children. However, methodological limitations in available epidemiological studies preclude clear determination of prevalence among older youth.[3]

In 2007, 2.2 million children and adolescents were taking medication for ADHD, far less than expected given disorder prevalence estimates of 5.4 million in the same age group.[2] This contradicts suggestions by some that ADHD medications are overprescribed.

Adult ADHD prevalence rates were at one time extrapolated from longitudinal studies of grown-up children previously diagnosed with the disorder. These suggested that more than half of ADHD-affected children have ongoing symptoms and related impairment as adults. In 2006, the National Comorbidity Survey Replication estimated the adult prevalence of ADHD at 4.4%.[4] A similar international study found a slightly lower but comparable rate.[5] These findings are consistent with, and provide support for, estimates suggested by longitudinal follow-up studies. Unlike generally episodic conditions such as mood and anxiety disorders, adults with ADHD typically have unremitting symptoms that require ongoing management.

Psychiatric Comorbidity

ADHD creates substantial risk for additional psychopathology (see Chapter 11). Over two thirds of children with ADHD have at least one additional psychiatric disorder and 18% have three or more other disorders.[6] The risk for having three or more additional disorders is higher in children from poorer families. Children with ADHD have increased rates of learning disabilities, oppositional defiant disorder, conduct disorder, depression, anxiety, and other conditions, compared with unaffected children (Fig. 3.1).

Adults with ADHD also demonstrate higher rates of co-occurring psychiatric disorders (Fig. 3.2). In particular, adults with ADHD have difficulties with other disorders of impulse control, including antisocial personality,

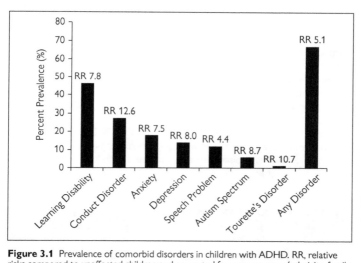

Figure 3.1 Prevalence of comorbid disorders in children with ADHD. RR, relative risks compared to unaffected children and corrected for age, sex, race/ethnicity, family structure, and household income. All differences significant, p <.05. (Adapted from Larson et al.[6])

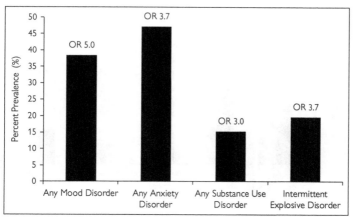

Figure 3.2 Past 12-month comorbidity of other psychiatric disorders in adults with ADHD. OR, odds ratio. All differences significant compared with non-ADHD comparisons, p <.05. (Adapted from Kessler et al.[4])

intermittent explosive disorder, and gambling, as well as increased lifetime histories of mood, anxiety, and substance use disorders.[4] Increased risks for substance use disorders and antisocial traits in adults with ADHD are generally mediated by a history of juvenile conduct disorder.

Although often unrecognized, ADHD similarly co-occurs at increased rates in individuals diagnosed with other emotional and behavioral disorders (Table 3.1). The degree to which untreated ADHD contributes to additional impairment and poorer outcomes in these patients has not been established.

Accidents, Risk Taking, and Medical Outcomes

Children with ADHD are more likely to have nonfatal accidental injuries, increased emergency room and hospital admissions, more major accidents, and higher rates of sexually transmitted disease (Fig. 3.3).[7] Older youth with ADHD have more motor vehicle accidents, traffic citations, and incidents of driving while intoxicated. Studies of children with ADHD followed as adults reveal increased rates of risky driving and sexual behaviors, increased nonalcohol substance use disorders and nicotine dependence, and increased difficulties with traffic accidents and speeding tickets (Fig. 3.4). Individuals

Table 3.1 Percentages of Patients with Other Psychiatric Conditions and Comorbid ADHD

Psychiatric Disorder	% With ADHD
Major depression	13%
Anxiety disorders	10%
Substance use disorders	11%
Impulse control disorders	12%

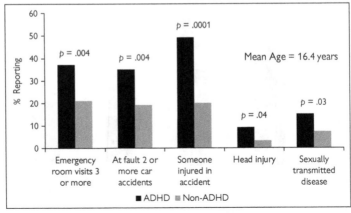

Figure 3.3 Medical outcomes with ADHD versus non-ADHD. (Adapted from Olazagasti et al.[7])

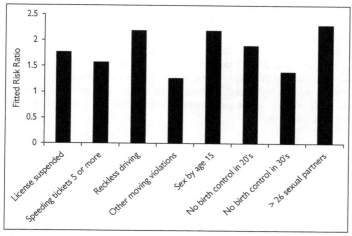

Figure 3.4 Increased risky behaviors in adults with ADHD compared with non-ADHD. All comparisons significant, $p < .05$. (Adapted from Olazagasti et al.[7])

with ADHD are more likely to have earlier initiation of sexual activity, more lifetime sexual partners, and decreased contraception use. These risks are particularly prominent in children with ADHD who also develop associated problems with conduct and antisocial personality disorder.

Functional Impairments

ADHD is associated over the life span with impairments in family, academic, social, and occupational functioning.[6] Families exhibit increased parental conflict and aggravation. Academic underperformance and other school-related problems are typical. Children with ADHD are almost 10 times more likely to have difficulties with making or keeping friends.[2] Childhood ADHD leads to greater occurrence of adolescent and adult criminal behaviors.[7] These risks are most evident in the third of ADHD-affected children who also develop secondary conduct disorder. Children with ADHD have higher rates of lifetime arrests, criminal convictions, and incarcerations. Adolescents with ADHD are more likely than typically developing youth to have spent time on probation or in jail, and to have been assigned by a court to a clinical social worker.

Adults with ADHD consistently demonstrate difficulties with academic and occupational achievement.[8] Those who enroll in college and succeed in obtaining degrees often require 5 to 6 years to complete their studies, compared with the usual 4 years. Increased substance abuse, early and risky sexual behavior, and poor adaptive skills often lead to personal instability with concomitant demoralization and low self-esteem.[7] It is unclear whether equal risk for these negative outcomes exists for women or those with a predominance of inattentive symptoms. Adults who seek treatment for school, work, or personal difficulties exhibit poor academic and occupational performance, dissatisfaction with friendships and intimate relationships, low self-esteem, substance abuse, and antisocial behaviors.[8] Employees with ADHD take more frequent sick days from work.[2] Other discrepancies in ADHD-affected adults include lower levels of education compared to cognitively matched peers, poor management of personal finances, more divorces and other relationship failures, and higher degrees of personal chaos.[8]

Economic Burden

Individual and social costs associated with ADHD are substantial and lasting.[9] The financial consequences of ADHD are borne by affected individuals, their families, and broader society in terms of lost productivity and income, health costs, educational failures, substance abuse, and increased criminality. Total estimated annual costs of ADHD in the United States in 2010 dollars range from $143 to $266 billion. Per-person costs are estimated to range from $621 to $2,720 for children and adolescents, and $137 to $4,120 for adults. Almost 75% of costs associated with ADHD are related to adults with ADHD or adult family members who miss work to take care of their affected children. Child and adolescent costs are mostly attributable to health care and education expense, while adult costs are mainly due to losses in income and productivity.

Average annual medical costs for children and adolescents with ADHD are three times higher than for typically developing youth.[10] Medical costs for non-ADHD family members of ADHD patients are more than double those in families without ADHD. These increased costs result from inpatient hospital expense, primary care visits, mental and behavioral health visits, and prescription medications, and are comparable to those seen with children suffering from other chronic medical conditions, such as asthma. Similarly, adults with ADHD have annual medical costs two to three times higher than matched non-ADHD comparisons.

Direct medical costs for the management of ADHD usually range from $1,000 to $5,000 per person annually.[9] This includes clinic visits, prescription medications, and other adjunctive therapies such as parent management training. It does not include additional expenses associated with academic accommodations, tutoring, or other specialized school services.

Additional indirect costs are borne by the parents of children and employers of adults.[9] Childhood ADHD increases the strain in parent–child relationships and heightens parental conflict. Parents of children with ADHD have 1.6 times as many claims for their own medical care compared with controls. Similarly, indirect costs due to parental disability and work absenteeism result from the need to miss work for direct child care, meeting with teachers, and bringing children to medical and other service appointments. On average, adults with ADHD are less productive at work and are more likely to take sick days or exhibit repeated absenteeism.

Adult professionals with ADHD who have obtained college degrees on average earn $40,000 less per year than similarly matched comparisons without the disorder.[11]

Criminal behaviors associated with ADHD create added societal economic burdens. Total costs for criminal behavior among juveniles is three times higher for youth with ADHD compared with controls.[10]

ADHD is associated with increased costs for management of other comorbid psychiatric and general medical conditions. One study demonstrated average increased costs of $358 per patient per year for management of depression, $258 for oppositional defiant disorder, $541 for bipolar disorder, $488 for anxiety, $868 for substance abuse, $198 for tics, and $247 for personality disorders.[10] Costs also increased for several general medication conditions, including $630 for respiratory illness, $670 for acute sinusitis, $972 for general injuries, and $507 for allergies. Whether these expenses can be reduced with aggressive ADHD management is not presently known and requires additional research.

References

1. Polanczyk G, Silva de Lima M. Horta BL, Biederman J, Rohde LA. The worldwide prevalence of ADHD: a systematic review and metaregression analysis. *Am J Psychiatry*. 2007;164:942–948.

2. Centers for Disease Control and Prevention. Increasing prevalence of parent-reported attention-deficit/hyperactivity disorder among children—United States, 2003 and 2007. *MMWR*. 2010;59:1439–1443.

3. Kessler RC, Avenevoli S, McLaughlin KA, et al. Lifetime co-morbidity of DSM-IV disorders in the US National Survey Replication Adolescent Supplement (NCS-A). *Psychol Med*. 2012;42:1997–2010.

4. Kessler RC, Adler L, Barkley R, et al. The prevalence and correlates of adult ADHD in the United States: results from the National Comorbidity Survey Replication. *Am J Psychiatry*. 2006;163:716–723.

5. Fayyad J, De Graaf R, Kessler R, et al. Cross-national prevalence and correlates of adult attention-deficit hyperactivity disorder. *BJP*. 2007;190:402–409.

6. Larson K, Russ SA, Kahn RS, Halfon N. Patterns of comorbidity, functioning, and service use for US children with ADHD, 2007. *Pediatrics*. 2011;127:462–470.

7. Olazagasti MA, Klein RG, Mannuzza S, et al. Does childhood attention-deficit/hyperactivity disorder predict risk-taking and medical illnesses in adulthood? *J Am Acad Child Adolesc Psychiatry*. 2013;52:153–162.

8. Barkley RA, Murphy KR, Smallish L, Fletcher K. Young adult outcomes of hyperactive children: adaptive functioning in major life activities. *J Am Acad Child Adolesc Psychiatry*. 2006;45:191–202.

9. Doshi JA, Hodgkins P, Kahle J, et al. Economic impact of childhood and adult attention-deficit/hyperactivity disorder in the United Stats. *J Am Acad Child Adolesc Psychiatry*. 2012;51:990–1002.

10. Matza LS, Paramore C, Prasad M. A review of the economic burden of ADHD. *Cost Eff Resour Alloc*. 2005;3:5.

11. Biederman J, Faraone SV. The effects of attention-deficit/hyperactivity disorder on employment and household income. *Med Gen Med*. 2006;8:12.

Further Reading

Nigg J. Attention-deficit/hyperactivity disorder and adverse health outcomes. *Clin Psychol Rev*. 2013;33:215–228.

Pelham WE, Foster EM, Robb JA. The economic impact of attention-deficit/hyperactivity disorder in children and adolescents. *Ambul Pediatr*. 2007;7:121–131.

Willcutt EG. The prevalence of DSM-IV attention-deficit/hyperactivity disorder: a meta-analytic review. *Neurotherapeutics*. 2012;9:490–499.

Chapter 4

Etiology and Neurobiology

> **Key Points**
>
> - The biological basis of ADHD is strongly evidenced in genetic and brain imaging studies.
> - ADHD is a complex trait likely to arise from the interactions of multiple genes and environmental factors.
> - Neuropsychological models emphasize deficits in executive function and reward pathways that likely represent dysfunction in multiple brain circuits.
> - Despite demonstrated biological difference in groups with and without ADHD, the disorder remains a behaviorally defined syndrome diagnosed by careful assessment of symptoms and clinical history, not by laboratory tests or brain imaging.

Evidence supporting the biological underpinnings of ADHD is of the strongest of any psychiatric disorder. Earliest conceptualizations of the disorder were informed by observations of behavioral sequelae of the influenza pandemic of 1917 that suggested both inattention and overactive behavior resulted from brain pathology (see Chapter 2). This preliminary view has evolved in tandem with other advances in neuroscience that demonstrate relationships between brain functioning, cognition, and behavior. ADHD remains a clinical syndrome defined by clinical criteria. However, a century of research reveals that ADHD is a complex, brain-based, neurodevelopmental disorder likely arising from the interplay of numerous social, developmental, environmental, and genetic risk factors (Fig. 4.1).[1]

Psychosocial Risk

Psychosocial factors such as parenting style, parental conflict, or family stress do not appear to be primary causes of ADHD. Although families with one or more ADHD-affected members often exhibit higher levels of conflict, this usually results from the parents' need to manage children's oppositional or other problematic behaviors. Decreases in parental conflict and stress typically follow successful management of ADHD symptoms.

Although not causal, psychosocial adversity appears to exacerbate the ADHD symptom severity and clinical presentation.[2] Risk factors include severe marital discord, low socioeconomic status, economic stress, large

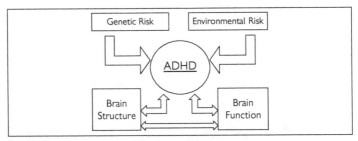

Figure 4.1 Biological basis of ADHD. (Adapted from Purper-Ouakil et al.[1])

family size, paternal criminality, maternal mental illness, abuse, and foster care placement. Aggregation of several risk factors rather than any one factor predicts greater ADHD severity. Conclusions about chronic family conflict, decreased family cohesion, and exposure to parental mental illness are difficult to untangle as these both result from ADHD and simultaneously appear to worsen ADHD-related difficulties.

ADHD-affected children often elicit parental interactions that compound rather than reduce the disorder's negative effects.[3] Children with ADHD are more frequently off task, more active, less compliant, and less responsive to discipline. Fathers of boys with ADHD are likely to be more demanding, aversive, and prone to use physical discipline. Mothers tend to be more disapproving, negative, inappropriately involved, and critical. This negative cycle of parent–child interaction worsens family, marital, and personal difficulties.

The negative effects of ineffective parenting are further exacerbated when one or both parents have ADHD. Children with ADHD have an estimated 30% chance of having at least one parent with the disorder. Parents with ADHD are often lax and inconsistent disciplinarians and have greater difficulty implementing recommended approaches to parenting.[3]

Prenatal and Perinatal Risk Factors

Prenatal factors associated with increased risk include maternal use of nicotine or alcohol during pregnancy, fetal exposure to other drugs or environmental factors, notably polychlorinated biphenyls (PCBs) and the insecticide DDT, and intrauterine growth delay.[4] Perinatal risks include poor maternal health, increased maternal age, prematurity, toxemia, preeclampsia, long labor, and fetal distress.[2] Particularly high risk is evident with births before 32 weeks gestation. Risk is even higher with births earlier than 28 weeks gestation, very low birth weight, particularly for newborns weighing 1,500 g (3 lb 5 oz) or less, and births later then 42 weeks gestation. Early postnatal risks include neonatal anoxia, seizures, and brain hemorrhage. Children exposed to early and severe institutional deprivation, such as seen in certain orphanages, often have ADHD symptoms, although these might be better correlated with attachment disorders.

Controversy persists regarding the relationship of maternal nicotine and alcohol consumption during gestation and subsequent ADHD risk.[2] Laboratory animal studies demonstrate increased hyperactivity with gestational nicotine exposure. However, since mothers with ADHD have increased risk for nicotine addiction and are less likely to quit or cut down use while pregnant, it remains unclear whether increased ADHD in their children results directly from in utero nicotine exposure or is due to inherited maternal genetic risks for the disorder. Preliminary research suggests that the link between maternal smoking and ADHD persists but is diminished after controlling for genetic and other environmental factors. This speaks to the public health benefit of reducing maternal nicotine and alcohol use during pregnancy.

Environmental Risk Factors

Elevated serum lead is associated with increased ADHD risk.[5] Symptom increases attributed to even miniscule lead levels are far lower than established safety thresholds. Direct causality, however, is difficult to demonstrate. Many individuals with elevated lead levels do not have ADHD, and lead exposure does not account for a substantial percentage of ADHD cases. Individuals with elevated lead levels frequently have other ADHD risk factors, including poverty and low parental educational attainment. Laboratory screening for serum lead is appropriate when clinical history raises concerns about possible lead ingestion. Chelation therapy can reduce ADHD symptoms in individuals positive for serum lead.

There are persistent assertions that dietary sugar, food additives, and/or deficits in vitamins and other micronutrients cause ADHD (see Chapter 13).[3] None of these claims has substantial support. Most studies examining a potential relationship between diet and ADHD suffer many methodological limitations, including very small sample sizes. Many parents have hard-held beliefs that chocolate or other foods high in refined sugar cause their children to be hyperactive due to an excess of energy. This opinion is not supported by controlled research and is not consistent with known physical effects of sugar ingestion. There is some evidence that artificial food additives might be associated with very small increased risk, but this might be true only in individuals with certain genotypes. If there is any causal relationship between diet and ADHD, the contribution of dietary factors to overall occurrence of ADHD is likely to be almost negligible.

ADHD Genetics

Initial interest in possible genetic underpinnings of ADHD emerged from family studies that began in the 1970s and demonstrated increased frequency of the disorder in first-degree relatives of ADHD-affected youth. Specifically, 20% to 30% of children with ADHD had at least one additional affected family member, suggesting a familial basis for the disorder.[6] Adoption studies revealed that adopted children with ADHD had similarly increased rates among their biological, but not adopted, relatives. Examinations of concordance rates in monozygotic and dizygotic twins consistently estimate that ADHD heritability approximates 74%, which suggests that 74% of the symptom variability in a population is due to genetic causes.[7] ADHD is about as heritable as height and is one of the most heritable psychiatric disorders (Fig. 4.2).

Early ADHD molecular genetics investigations were influenced by the idea that common disorders were caused by common genetic variants.[6] These studies were typically case-control and family-based investigations of candidate genes that were selected based on known targets and metabolic pathways of stimulant medications proven useful in ADHD treatment. Most emphasized allele variants in the dopamine and norepinephrine transmitter systems. There was initially great excitement surrounding two dopamine system variants, the variable number tandem repeat (VNTR) polymorphism found in the 3' untranslated region (UTR) region of the dopamine transporter (SLC6A3) and the 7-repeat allele of the 48-base pair VNTR found in exon 3 of the dopamine D4 receptor (DRD4). Other candidate genes also showed positive associations. However, findings from many of these early studies were not replicated in later investigations and were often limited by false-positive results, small sample sizes, and failures to consider population differences. Meta-analyses confirm positive findings for several candidate genes, but none of these is causal for ADHD and none, either alone or in combination, predicts substantial risk for the disorder.[6]

Genetic linkage studies in families with multiple affected members were conducted to assess cosegregation of genetic markers that could suggest certain genomic regions with high probability of harboring risk genes. Linkage studies examine the entire genome and do not require preconceived

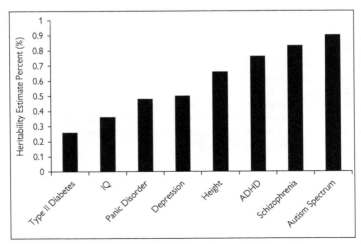

Figure 4.2 Heritability of ADHD and other complex traits. (Adapted from Purper-Ouakil et al.[1])

hypotheses about particular genes. These studies are limited to finding genes of larger effect, specifically genes that can account for more than 10% of symptom variance. A meta-analysis of seven ADHD linkage studies identified one significant peak on the long arm of chromosome 16, but no genes in that region have been implicated in candidate gene investigations.[8]

Genome-wide association studies (GWAS) compare single-nucleotide polymorphisms (SNPs) across the genome in individuals with and without disorders. Increased frequencies of particular SNPs identify genomic regions that likely contain genes related to the disorder of interest. Due to the high number of SNP comparisons, very stringent significance levels ($p < 10^{-8}$) are required to minimize false-positive findings. In initial ADHD GWAS, no findings attained statistical significance, but trends implicated multiple regions containing genes involved in directing cell architecture and communication.[6] A related GWAS of multiple psychiatric disorders identified four genomic regions likely to harbor common risk alleles for ADHD, depression, bipolar disorder, autism spectrum disorder, and schizophrenia.[9]

GWAS failed to support the idea that ADHD is substantially caused by common genetic variants or major risk genes. More recent studies suggest that individuals with ADHD have higher numbers of rare copy number variants (CNVs) across their genomes compared with unaffected individuals.[10] CNVs are insertion or deletion mutations that persist in the genome over time. Some CNVs associated with ADHD involve genes that regulate learning, behavior, synaptic transmission, and neural development, but overall CNV burden appears to be more important for ADHD risk than which genes are affected. CNVs might account for a substantial proportion of ADHD heritability in some families, but given that the variants are by definition rare they do not explain substantial overall population risk.

Gene–Environment Interactions

There is growing appreciation of the extent to which interactions between genetic and environmental factors increase disease risk. Although both genetic and environmental ADHD risk factors are identified, none is causal and many individuals with them do not develop the disorder. Evidence suggests that underlying ADHD genetic risks have greater expression in the context of high environmental adversity and are attenuated with increased psychosocial stability.

Several small studies suggest that specific gene–environment interactions are causal for ADHD.[6] One study demonstrated that maternal smoking during pregnancy was associated with increased risk for subsequent ADHD only when the child had specific risk alleles, specifically the 7-repeat of the *DRD4* exon III VNTR or the 10-repeat of the *SCL6A3* 3' UTR VNTR. Children lacking these exhibited much lower ADHD rates regardless of whether their mothers smoked. Similarly, it has been suggested that increased ADHD risk from certain food additives is influenced by the presence or absence of variants in histaminergic and dopaminergic genes. If validated in large samples, an increased understanding of gene–environment interactions and ADHD risk raises the possibility of primary prevention or symptom reduction through targeted environmental interventions for those with increased genetic risk.

Brain Imaging

Brain imaging is not useful or appropriate for ADHD diagnosis. There is a great range of variability and overlap in individuals with and without the disorder, such that imaging studies lack the predictive power that is necessary for a diagnostic test. Nonetheless, research on groups with and without ADHD has consistently demonstrated measurable differences in brain structure and function that provide a basis for understanding areas of brain dysfunction associated with the disorder.

Structural imaging studies using computerized tomography (CT) and magnetic resonance imaging (MRI) consistently find evidence of brain abnormalities, most commonly smaller total brain and white matter volumes with particular decreases in frontal cortex, cerebellum, and subcortical structures.[2] Caudate nucleus differences seem to disappear by adolescence. Differences in other brain structures appear fixed. Normalization in areas such as the parietal cortex and hippocampus are associated with symptom reduction, whereas ongoing volume loss is typically seen with symptom persistence. Longitudinal studies suggest that ADHD-affected groups have parallel but delayed patterns of brain development, with approximately 3-year delays in cortical maturation.[11] This suggests that early genetic and environmental effects on brain development are nonprogressive and stable.

Positron emission tomography (PET) in adult parents of children with ADHD revealed decreased glucose metabolism in the premotor and superior prefrontal cortices.[12] Studies using single-photon emission computerized tomography (SPECT) in ADHD diagnosed adults found decreased perfusion and underactivation in prefrontal regions, consistent with measured executive function deficits, as well as striatal regions.[12] Adult radioligand binding studies revealed decreased blood flow and increased density of dopamine transporters (DATs) in striatal regions.[12] Functional MRI (fMRI) studies in children and adolescents showed patterns of hypoactivation with ADHD, primarily in frontostriatal and parietal areas.[13]

Early imaging findings emphasized abnormalities in discrete brain regions and prefrontal-striatal circuits. More recently, the research emphasis has shifted toward examining patterns of dysfunction and altered connectivity across multiple neuronal systems that involve both higher level cognitive and sensorimotor processes (Fig. 4.3).[13] ADHD is associated with abnormal activation in large-scale brain systems. Children with ADHD exhibit hypoactivation in brain regions associated with executive function and attention, specifically the frontoparietal and ventral attentional networks, respectively, and hyperactivation in the default, ventral attentional and somatomotor networks. Adults demonstrate hypoactivation in the frontoparietal and hyperactivation in the visual, dorsal attention, and default networks.

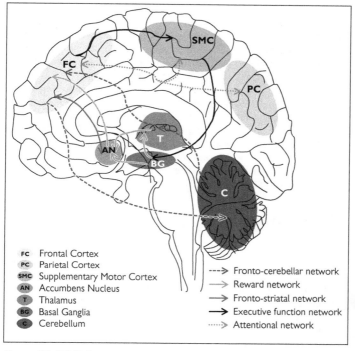

Figure 4.3 ADHD functional circuits. (Adapted from Purper-Ouakil et al.[1])

Neuropsychological Models

Neuropsychological tests identify patterns of cognitive dysfunction in ADHD that are often consistent with brain imaging abnormalities.[14] As with neuro-imaging, neuropsychological tests detect group effects that are not helpful in making ADHD diagnoses due to the high degree of variability exhibited by affected and unaffected individuals. Neuropsychological findings provide a basis for several models that help elucidate dysfunctional brain processes associated with the disorder. Abnormalities in brain function identified by neuropsychological testing have been proposed as ADHD endophenotypes, that is, more homogeneous subgroups within the broader *DSM*-defined behavioral syndrome that are attributable to more easily identified genetic underpinnings.

One popular neuropsychological model suggests that ADHD arises from primary deficits in executive functions (EFs), generally defined as cognitive processes that support appropriate problem-solving skills aimed toward achieving future goals.[15] Specifically, EFs maintain information about possible choices in working memory and facilitate integration with other relevant information from the current environmental context in order to make optimal choices in a given situation. EF deficits in ADHD include working memory, response inhibition, and general weaknesses in executive control. EF processes are largely functions of the prefrontal lobes, which are implicated further with behavioral hyperactivity, impulsivity, and inattention. Impaired EF appears to play an important role in the complex neuropsychology of ADHD, but it does not adequately explain all cases of the disorder.

The dual-pathway model of ADHD suggests that inattention and EF deficits result from impaired prefrontal-striatal circuits, while hyperactivity results from frontal-limbic dysfunctions that regulate motivation and reward response.[1] Another model proposes that impaired signaling in the prefrontal cortex leads to failures in detecting differences between actual and expected environmental inputs, which results in inappropriate behavioral responses. Ongoing work is required to elucidate specific relationships between ADHD symptoms and dysfunction in specific neural networks.

Clinical Implications

Our understanding of ADHD neurobiology provides biological validation of the disorder and reduces social stigma that results from those who deny the legitimacy of the condition or argue that it is merely a relative social construct. Increased knowledge about biological mechanisms associated with ADHD and related cognitive and behavioral impairment provides a foundation for development of new medication and psychosocial treatment strategies, as well as the targeting of specific interventions designed for optimized treatment of individual patients.

References

1. Purper-Ouakil D, Ramoz N, Lepagnol-Bestel A, Gorwood P, Simonneau M. Neurobiology of attention deficit/hyperactivity disorder. *Pediatr Res.* 2011;69:69R-76R.

2. Spencer T, Biederman J, Mick E. Attention-deficit/hyperactivity disorder: diagnosis, lifespan, comorbidities, and neurobiology. *J Pediatr Psychol.* 2007;32:631–642.

3. Daley D. Attention deficit hyperactivity disorder: a review of the essential facts. *Child Care Health Dev.* 2006;32:193–204.

4. Banerjee TD, Middleton F, Faraone SV. Environmental risk factors for attention-deficit/hyperactivity disorder. *Acta Paediatr.* 2007;96:1269–1274.

5. Nigg JT, Nikolas M, Mark Knottnerus M, Cavanagh K, Friderici K. Confirmation and extension of association of blood lead with attention-deficit/hyperactivity disorder (ADHD) and ADHD symptom domains at population-typical exposure levels. *J Child Psychol Psychiatry.* 2010;51:58–65.

6. Faraone SV, Mick E. Molecular genetics of attention deficit hyperactivity disorder. *Psychiatr Clin N Am.* 2010;33:159–180.

7. Faraone SV, Doyle AE. The nature and heritability of attention-deficit/hyperactivity disorder. *Child Adolesc Psychiatr Clin N Am.* 2001;10:299–316.

8. Zhou K, Dempfle A, Arcos-Burgos M, et al. Meta-analysis of genome-side linkage scans of attention deficit hyperactivity disorder. *Am J Med Genet B Neuropyschiatr Genet.* 2008;t147B:1392–1398.

9. Cross-Disorder Group of the Psychiatric Genomics Consortium. Genetic relationships between five psychiatric disorders estimated from genome-wide SNPs. *Nat Genet.* 2013;45:984–994.

10. Yang L, Neale BM, Liu L, et al. Polygenic transmission and complex neuro-developmental network for attention deficit hyperactivity disorder: genome wide association study of both common and rare variants. *Am J Med Gen B Neuropyschiatr Genet.* 2013;162B:419–430.

11. Shaw P, Eckstrand K, Sharp W, et al. Attention-deficit/hyperactivity disorder is characterized by a delay in cortical maturation. *Proc Natl Acad Sci USA.* 2007;104:19649–19654.

12. Cubilla A, Rubia K. Structural and functional brain imaging in adults with attention-deficit/hyperactivity disorder. *Expert Rev Neurother.* 2010;10:603–620.

13. Cortese S, Kelly C, Chabernaud C, et al. Towards systems neuroscience of ADHD: a meta-analysis of 55 fMRI studies. *Am J Psychiatry.* 2012;169:1038–1055.

14. Tripp G, Wickens JR. Neurobiology of ADHD. *Neuropharmacol.* 2009;57:579–589.

15. Willcutt EG, Doyle AE, Nigg JT, Faraone SV, Pennington BF. Validity of executive function theory of attention-deficit/hyperactivity disorder: a meta-analytic review. *Biol Psychiatry.* 2005;57:1336–1346.

Further Reading

Sonuga-Barke EJ. The dual pathway model of AD/HD: an elaboration of neuro-developmental characteristics. *Neuro Sci Biobev Rev.* 2003;27:593–604.

Weyandt L, Swentosky A, Gudmundsdottir BG. Neuroimaging and ADHD, PET, DTI findings, and methodological limitations. *Dev Neuropsychol.* 2013;38:211–225.

Chapter 5

Diagnostic Criteria

Key Points

- ADHD is diagnosed on the basis of persistent difficulties from symptoms of inattention and/or hyperactivity-impulsivity that occur to a greater degree than expected for an individual's developmental level.
- Diagnosis is based on clinical criteria as currently defined in the *DSM-5*.
- *DSM-5* criteria incorporate a developmental perspective that recognizes symptom changes and thresholds for diagnosis as individuals become older adolescents and adults.

While much research demonstrates its biological correlates (see Chapter 4), ADHD remains a clinically defined syndrome diagnosed on the basis of structured clinical criteria. ADHD is classified in the Neurodevelopmental Disorders section of the *Diagnostic and Statistical Manual of Mental Disorders*, fifth edition (*DSM-5*), which reflects its initial presentation in childhood and frequent co-occurrence with other early-onset brain-based disorders. ADHD diagnostic criteria are summarized in Box 5.1

Historical Perspectives

Regardless of what it has been called, developmentally inappropriate levels of inattention, impulsivity, and hyperactivity have always defined ADHD (see Chapter 2). The *Diagnostic and Statistical Manual of Mental Disorders*, second edition (*DSM-II*) broadly characterized the hyperkinetic reaction of childhood (or adolescence) in those youth who exhibited difficulties due to overactivity, restlessness, distractibility, and short attention span. *DSM-II* largely viewed hyperkinetic reaction as a disorder of younger children with the expectation that these behaviors diminished by adolescence.

The *Diagnostic and Statistical Manual of Mental Disorders*, third edition (*DSM-III*) provided the first elucidation of specific symptom sets, which were organized into three areas of inattention, impulsivity, and hyperactivity. A panel of experts in childhood psychopathology proposed symptoms based on their own clinical and research experience, but there were no attempts to validate these diagnostic criteria. In *DSM-III*, the diagnosis of attention-deficit disorder with hyperactivity (ADDH) required a minimum of three of five inattentive, three of six impulsive, and two of six hyperactive symptoms, while a diagnosis of attention-deficit disorder without hyperactivity (ADDWO)

Box 5.1 Summary of ADHD Diagnosis Criteria

According to the criteria in the *DSM-5*, persistent impaired behavior for a minimum of 6 months that exceeds what is expected for an individual's developmental level and is characterized by at least 6 of 9 inattentive and/or 6 of 9 hyperactive-impulsive symptoms is required in order to make an ADHD diagnosis. If the patient is 17 or older, only 5 of 9 symptoms are required.

The patient also must show some history of symptoms before age 12 and at least several symptoms must occur in more than one setting (e.g., home, school, social relations, work, recreational activities, etc.). The symptoms also must result in clinically meaningful impairment in social, academic, or occupational functioning; and the symptoms must not have occurred due to schizophrenia or other psychotic illness and cannot be better explained by conditions such as mood, anxiety, personality, or substance use disorders.

required only the minimum number of inattentive and impulsive symptoms. The revised *DSM-III* (*DSM-III-R*) replaced the three separate symptom sets with a single list of 14 symptoms, required a minimum of eight symptoms for the diagnosis, and eliminated any distinction between individuals with and without hyperactivity.

The single symptom list in *DSM-III-R* suggested that ADHD existed along a single dimension, instead of the three originally conceived in *DSM-III*. Subsequent analysis of several data sets revealed that ADHD appeared to comprise two symptom dimensions, the inattentive and hyperactive-impulsive. Some investigators voiced surprise that impulsive symptoms were associated with hyperactivity, and not inattention, as originally thought. Recognition of the two-dimensional structure of ADHD symptoms informed the conduct of clinical field trials designed to provide an empirical basis for a revised classification system in the *Diagnostic and Statistical Manual of Mental Disorders*, fourth edition (*DSM-IV*).

Symptoms

DSM-5 retains the same set of 18 ADHD symptoms used in *DSM-IV*, nine inattentive (Table 5.1) and nine hyperactive/impulsive (Table 5.2). In field trials conducted for *DSM-IV*, the clinical utility of potential symptoms derived from *DSM-III, DSM-III-R*, and *ICD-10* was assessed in several hundred pediatric patients ages 4–17 years.[1] Clinicians participating in the trial designated which of these proposed symptoms characterized their own patients diagnosed with ADHD. Investigators further assessed the correlation of proposed symptoms with parent and teacher impairment ratings. *DSM-IV* included those symptoms that best differentiated patients with ADHD from other disorders and also best correlated with parent and teacher ratings of impairment.

Table 5.1 ADHD Inattentive Symptoms

	Younger Individuals	Older Individuals
1	Fails to notice details, makes careless errors	Careless or inaccurate work
2	Trouble maintaining attention	Trouble staying focused on boring work, mind wanders, difficulty with sustained reading
3	Appears not to listen even when spoken to directly	Difficulty focusing on what people say, even when addressed directly
4	Trouble completing tasks or following through on instructions	Has difficulty finishing tasks, easily sidetracked
5	Difficulty with organization	Procrastinates, trouble completing tasks in order, messy, misses deadlines
6	Avoids activities that require sustained attention	Delays or avoids work or activities that are boring or repetitive
7	Loses or misplaces things	Often misplaces things required at work, home, or other activities
8	Distracted easily by extraneous stimuli	Distracted by surrounding noises or other activities, or by unrelated thoughts
9	Forgets easily	Trouble remembering appointments and other obligations

Table 5.2 ADHD Hyperactive-Impulsive Symptoms

	Younger Individuals	Older Individuals
1	Frequently fidgets, taps hands or feet, squirms when seated	Often restless or fidgety
2	Frequently gets out of seat	Often leaves seats at meetings and other times seating is required
3	Runs and climbs when inappropriate	Feels internally restless
4	Unable to play quietly	Often louder than appropriate for a given situation
5	Frequently "on the go" as if "driven by a motor"	Has trouble unwinding or relaxing, always needs something to do
6	Talks to excess	Talks too much in social situations
7	Blurts out answers before questions are completed	Finishes others' sentences or answers questions before they are finished
8	Trouble waiting turn or in line	Difficulty standing in line or waiting turn
9	Frequently interrupts or intrudes	Interrupts others' conversations and activities, intrudes into what others are doing

DSM-IV ADHD symptoms have proven useful in extensive research and clinical practice. The decision to retain *DSM-IV* symptoms in *DSM-5* allows continuity in clinical diagnosis and the application of past research. A major shortcoming of the *DSM-IV* ADHD field trial was its sole focus on school-age children. Few older adolescents and no adults participated. Whether *DSM-IV* symptoms were developmentally representative of older patients had never been demonstrated. Some symptoms, such as "runs and climbs excessively" and "has difficulty playing quietly," were irrelevant in older persons. Although *DSM-5* includes the same set of *DSM-IV* ADHD symptoms, the text discussion expands consideration of how they expressed in older individuals. This approach places symptom assessment in a more appropriate developmental context. Regardless of a person's age, the diagnosis depends on symptom frequency and severity that exceeds what is expected for the individual's developmental level.

Diagnostic Thresholds

There has been ongoing debate about whether ADHD is a categorical or dimensional disorder. In a categorical disorder, individuals either have or do not have the condition. Examples are pneumonia, otitis media, enuresis, and anorexia nervosa. In a dimensional disorder, symptoms or laboratory values exist in a continuum within the population, and one end of the distribution is associated with increased risk for morbidity or other impairments. Examples are blood pressure, cholesterol, intelligence, and possibly mood and anxiety symptoms. Frequently within psychiatric classification, neither approach is completely satisfactory in defining various conditions.

Symptoms of inattention, impulsivity, and hyperactivity clearly exist across the population. Many have argued that these symptoms are quite normal for certain ages and circumstances. In *DSM-IV*, cutoffs of six symptoms in either the inattentive or hyperactive/impulsive dimension were based on field trial data demonstrating that 50% of patients identified by clinicians as having ADHD had six or more symptoms.[1] The six-symptom cutoff also correlated strongly with parent and teacher impairment ratings. Furthermore, this cutoff falls approximately two standard deviations above the mean and at the 92nd percentile for total number of symptoms for school-age children.

Many studies, including genetic and imaging studies, have demonstrated significant differences in individuals with and without ADHD based on meeting or failing to meet the categorical cutoff of six symptoms (see Chapter 4). Other studies, particularly brain imaging studies, have demonstrated incremental differences that correlate with increasing symptom number along a dimension of symptom number, regardless of a discrete cutoff.

The mean number of ADHD symptoms exhibited at any given age decreases over time.[2] Requiring six symptoms for diagnosis in adults meant that older patients had numbers of symptoms three to four standard deviations greater than expected for their age, a much higher threshold than required in children. Studies demonstrated that adults with as few as four inattentive symptoms had significant impairments relative to their peers. This suggested that the *DSM-IV* requirement for six symptoms was overly restrictive and failed to identify considerable numbers of older patients with meaningful levels of clinical impairment.[3]

DSM-5 introduced a level of developmental sensitivity to the symptom threshold required for diagnosis. The first criterion for ADHD continues to require a minimum of six of nine inattentive and/or six of nine specified hyperactive-impulsive symptoms for diagnosis in children and younger adolescents. However, only five symptoms in either category are sufficient when patients are 17 years or older. This modification is consistent with the requirement for a persistent pattern of inattention and/or hyperactivity-impulsivity that is developmentally inappropriate and meaningfully interferes with development or functioning.

Age of Onset

Some history of ADHD symptoms history prior to age 12 is required for diagnosis. This represents a change from previous *DSM* editions. In the early 1980s, investigators decided to require an age of symptom onset prior to 7 years as a means to create more homogeneous research groups and ensure that clinical subjects were suffering from a developmental, that is, early-onset, disorder. *DSM-III* incorporated the age of 7 onset criterion without any particular scientific basis. *DSM-IV* further complicated matters in requiring that clinically meaningful impairment as well as symptoms had to be evident before age 7.[4]

Recognition of the difficulties that arose from attempts to apply this criterion retrospectively, particularly in adults, led to changing the required age of onset from younger than age 7 to younger than age 12. The *DSM-IV* field trial itself found a significant number of individuals assessed as having ADHD who failed to have an age of onset or associated impairment prior to age 7.[4] For those with the predominately inattentive subtype, 15% and 43% failed to have symptoms and impairment, respectively, by the age cutoff. Other studies showed that no differences in patterns of comorbidity or impairment were evident between those who did and did not report early onset. Adult studies, which generally relied on retrospective determination of age of onset, had similar findings. As with children in the *DSM-IV* field trial, individuals with early versus late onset had no differences in functional impairment, age, education, psychological adjustment, or neuropsychiatric testing.[5] Other studies suggested that virtually all adults otherwise diagnosed with ADHD report age of onset prior to age 12. Changing this criterion to require age of onset prior to 12 resulted in virtually no additional persons being assigned the diagnosis.[6]

A related issue is the degree to which it is feasible to expect adults to report reliably on childhood symptoms and impairments.[3] In a longitudinal study of school-age children diagnosed with ADHD, adult participants were asked to recall the onset of their childhood symptoms and related difficulties. Just over half accurately recounted an onset of symptoms prior to age 7. On average, the group recalled an age of onset 4 year later than described by their parents in real time. This suggests that retrospectively adults tend to report that problems related to ADHD emerged several years later than described by their parents when they were children.

The unlinking of impairment from the age of onset criterion reflects growing recognition that some individuals with ADHD, particularly those with higher intelligence or stronger support systems, are able to compensate for the disorder and not exhibit meaningful difficulties. At times, clinically

CHAPTER 5 **Diagnostic Criteria**

significant impairment does not emerge until individuals face increased demands of higher education or employment. In these cases, some history of symptoms prior to age 12 is required, but the diagnosis is dependent on current impairment and not retrospective recall of childhood difficulties.

Domains of Clinical Impairment

A history of ADHD symptoms and associated difficulties should be evident in at least two settings. Common areas of impairment in children include family life, school, and peer relationships. Additionally, older youth and adults typically have problems with employment, driving, accidental injuries, general health choices, and interpersonal conflicts. Some individuals, particularly adults, acknowledge impairment in only one area, while exhibiting restrictive life choices that suggest broader difficulties. Examples might be a single adult who lives alone and denies difficulties outside of work, a chronically underemployed actress waiting to be cast in a role, or a successful businessman threatened with a divorce. It is expected that impairments in multiple areas should be evident over an individual's life history, even though an individual might only admit to one current area of difficulty. Clinicians should assess functional impairment in relation to social norms exhibited by the individual patient's reference group.

Differential Diagnosis

ADHD is not diagnosed if symptoms occur solely during the course of schizophrenia or another psychotic disorder, or if symptoms are better explained by another mental disorder. The previous exclusion for pervasive developmental disorders, now subsumed under autism spectrum disorder, has been eliminated. An individual with autism spectrum disorder, intellectual disability, or other developmental disorder should also be diagnosed with ADHD if he or she meets criteria, with the caveat that symptom frequency and severity must exceed what is expected generally for that person's developmental level, not chronological age.

Many mental disorders share ADHD features. The clinician must determine if symptoms are better explained by other disorders or if other disorders are comorbid with ADHD. Often a deciding feature in support of ADHD is a persistent history of difficulties with inattentive and/or hyperactive-impulsive symptoms that precede and continue outside of any discrete episode of mood, anxiety, or behavioral difficulties. When symptoms are not persistent, they are more likely to represent conditions other than ADHD. Other disorders should be diagnosed as comorbid with ADHD when both sets of criteria are met.

Specifiers

DSM-IV created a great emphasis on ADHD subtypes. Patients with sufficient symptoms in both the inattentive and hyperactive-impulsive categories were deemed to have the Combined subtype. Those with six or more inattentive but fewer than six hyperactive-impulsive were categorized by the predominately Inattentive subtype. Those with six or more hyperactive-impulsive symptoms but fewer than six inattentive were categorized as the predominately Hyperactive-impulsive subtype.

DSM-IV subtypes posed several difficulties.[3] Subtypes were not stable over time, and individuals often manifested different subtypes at different ages. Genetic studies showed that while ADHD was highly heritable, subtypes were not. Subtypes had no predictive value for treatment response.

DSM-5 eliminated subtypes and replaced them with specifiers that describe clinical presentation in the preceding 6 months. Patients meeting diagnostic thresholds for both inattentive and hyperactive-impulsive symptoms are specified as having the Combined presentation. Those meeting the diagnostic threshold only for inattentive or hyperactive-impulsive symptoms are specified as having, respectively, either the Inattentive or Hyperactive-impulsive presentation. Use of these specifiers allows greater descriptive characterization of individual patients. Whether or not this added specification has any other value is as yet unknown.

As with many disorders, ADHD severity can be specified based on the number of presenting symptoms. *Mild* ADHD is specified when few, if any, symptoms are present in excess of what is required and if there is no more than minor functional difficulties. *Severe* ADHD is specified when many symptoms in excess of what is required are present, or if there is marked functional impairment in one or more settings. *Moderate* ADHD is specified when symptoms and impairment fall somewhere between "mild" and "severe."

ADHD can be specified "in partial remission" when a patient previously met full criteria, currently has fewer than the necessary symptom number for full diagnosis, but continues to exhibit clinically meaningful impairment due to remaining symptoms.

Other Specified and Unspecified ADHD

Individuals who suffer clinically significant impairment due to ADHD symptoms but do not meet full diagnostic criteria can be assigned the diagnosis "other specified ADHD." The diagnosis should then specify the reason full criteria were not met, such as "other specified ADHD with insufficient inattentive and hyperactive-impulsive symptoms." If a clinician chooses not to specify which criteria are lacking, it is acceptable to assign a diagnosis of "unspecified ADHD."

References

1. Lahey BB, Applegate B, McBurnett K, et al. DSM-IV field trials for attention deficit hyperactivity disorder in children and adolescents. *Am J Psychiatry.* 1994;151:1673–1685.

2. Biederman J, Mick E, Faraone SV. Age-dependent decline of symptoms of attention deficit hyperactivity disorder: impact of remission definition and symptom type. *Am J Psychiatry.* 2000;157:818–818.

3. McGough JJ, Barkley RA. Diagnostic controversies in adult attention deficit hyperactivity disorder. *Am J Psychiatry.* 2004;161:1948–1956.

4. Applegate B, Lahey BB, Hart EL, et al. Validity of the age-of-onset criterion for ADHD: a report from the DSM-IV field trials. *J Am Acad Child Adolesc Psychiatry.* 1997;36:1211–1221.

5. Faraone SV, Biederman J, Spencer T, et al. Diagnosing adult attention deficit hyperactivity disorder: are late onset and subthreshold diagnoses valid? *Am J Psychiatry.* 2006;163:1720–1729.

6. Polanczyk G, Caspi A, Houts R, Kollins SH, Rohde LA, Moffitt TE. Implications of extending the ADHD age-of-onset criterion to 12: results from a prospectively studied birth cohort. *J Am Acad Child Adolesc Psychiatry.* 2010;49:210–216.

Further Reading

American Psychiatric Association. *Diagnostic and Statistical Manual of Mental Disorders* (5th ed.). Arlington, VA: American Psychiatric Association, 2013.

Solanto MV, Wasserstein J, Marks DJ, Mitchell KJ. Diagnosis of ADHD in adults: what is the appropriate DSM-5 symptom threshold for hyperactivity/impulsivity? *J Attent Disord.* 2012;16:631–634.

Willcutt EG, Nigg JT, Pennington BF, et al. Validity of DSM-IV attention deficit/hyperactivity disorder symptom dimensions and subtypes. *J Abnorm Psychol.* 2012:121:991–1010.

Chapter 6

Assessment

Key Points

- ADHD is a behavioral syndrome diagnosed on the basis of clinical criteria.
- ADHD assessment relies on careful integration of clinical information derived from a wide variety of sources.
- Comorbidity is typical and should be considered in any ADHD evaluation.
- ADHD is not diagnosed with neuropsychological tests, computerized tests of attention, laboratory measures, EEG profiles, or brain imaging.

ADHD should be assessed in any child or adolescent exhibiting academic or behavioral difficulties or any adult with long-standing problems due to inattention or distractibility. The diagnosis reflects a clinical picture that generally begins before or during grade school, persists over time, manifests in different settings, and is associated with clinically significant impairment in a range of life activities, including family, school, social, and occupational functioning.

ADHD is most reliably assessed by careful review and integration of clinical information obtained from multiple sources. These include parent, teacher, and other third-party reports, patient self-report rating scales, past psychiatric and medical histories, educational and occupational records, clinical interviews, direct observation, and, in some cases, psychoeducational testing (Fig. 6.1). Diagnosis cannot rely on any individual rating scale or bit of clinical information.

For children and adolescents, the most critical aspect of the evaluation is a face-to-face interview with one or both parents and the child. For adults, the patient is usually the primary informant, but family members, partners, employers, and others can provide helpful supplemental data. In all cases, review and documentation of ADHD symptoms as defined by *DSM-5* is paramount (see Chapter 5). ADHD is a clinical syndrome. Although neuropsychological testing can be valuable in assessing particular cases, ADHD is not diagnosed on the basis of any distinct neuropsychological profile. There is no scientific justification for claiming to diagnose ADHD on the basis of other laboratory studies, computerized tests of attention, electroencephalography (EEG), or other brain imaging methods.

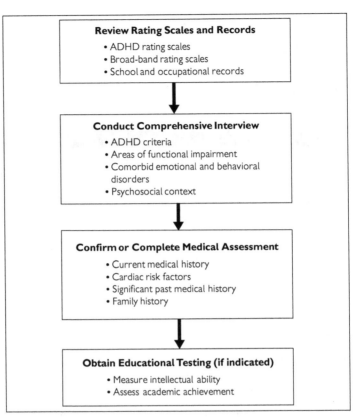

Figure 6.1 ADHD assessment.

Rating Scales and Record Review

Rating scales provide easily reviewed clinical data that supplement information obtained during the face-to-face interview. Developmental questionnaires and behavioral rating scales can be sent to families when the initial assessment is scheduled. For younger patients, rating scales are usually obtained from parents and teachers. For older individuals, self-reports, as well as ratings from spouses, partners, employers, family members, and friends, are useful. Ideally, completed rating scales are available at the intake visit.

Numerous ADHD rating scales are available and used routinely both in initial assessments and documenting treatment response (Table 6.1). It is unnecessary for parents, teachers, or patients to complete multiple ADHD-specific scales, as most are based primarily on *DSM* symptoms. Most currently available scales reference *DSM-IV*, but these remain useful as symptoms remain

Table 6.1 ADHD Rating Scales

Rating Scale	How Obtained
Children and Adolescents	
ADHD Rating Scale-IV (ADHD-RS)	Purchase book and copy: DuPaul GJ, Power TJ, Anastopoulos AD, Reid R. ADHD Rating Scale—IV (for Children and Adolescents). Guilford Press.
Brown Attention Deficit Disorder Scales	Purchase: PsychCorp Pearson. www.psychcorp. peasrsonassessments.com
Conners, 3rd Edition Rating Scales	Purchase: Multi-Health Systems, Inc. www.mhs.com
Swanson Nolan and Pelham (SNAP-IV) Teacher and Parent Rating Scales	Free download: www.adhd.net
Vanderbilt Teacher and Parent Rating Scales	Free download: www.nihcq.org/toolkit
Adults	
Barkley Adult ADHD Rating Scale-IV (BAARS-IV)	Purchase and copy: Barkley RA. Barkley's Adult ADHD Rating Scale IV (BAARS-IV). Guilford Press.
Brown Attention Deficit Disorder Scales	Purchase: PsychCorp Pearson. www.psychcorp. peasrsonassessments.com
Conners' Adult ADHD Rating Scales	Purchase: Multi-Health Systems, Inc. www.mhs.com
World Health Organization Adult ADHD Self Report Scale (ASRS)	Download: www.webdoc.nyumc.org/nyumc_d6/files/ psych_adhd_screener.pdf

unchanged in *DSM-5*. At times, individuals have their own biases in completing rating scales and the clinician must carefully balance and assess the implications of conflicting reports. Other general rating scales, such as the Child Behavior Checklist (CBCL) or Symptom Checklist-90 Revised (SCL-90R), are not specific for any diagnosis but are frequently used to obtain broad measures of psychological functioning and impairment to supplement ADHD-specific ratings.

In addition to ratings scales, it is important to review any available school records, standardized test results, employment records, and previous educational or psychological test reports. Clinicians can quickly review these records and integrate them with other available data.

Clinical Interview

In younger patients, parents are the primary informants. Interviewing third parties is less important with older patients and not routine with adults. Except with very young children, some portion of the initial assessment should be conducted alone with the patient. Having individual time with children apart from parents can help in assessment of ADHD symptoms, social relatedness, and other psychiatric conditions, as well as provide a foundation for ongoing treatment. Individual time with older children and adolescents is essential for building trust and discussing sensitive topics such as sexual activity and illicit substance use. Adult patients, at times, will ask to include partners or other adults in their evaluation. It is usually best to allow this only after the initial private interview is completed.

Approaches to assessment might differ depending on the clinician's specialty training or practice setting. Primary care physicians generally have less time for initial evaluations but better access to past medical history, knowledge of the family, and patient's community. Specialists, such as psychiatrists, neurologists, and psychologists, usually have longer initial visits and are better able to assess psychiatric comorbidities but have less access to medical records. In all cases, routine use of rating scales completed before the evaluation and reviewed during the office visit greatly facilitates efficient clinical management.

In research settings, diagnosis is usually based on structured or semistructured reviews of *DSM* symptoms using standard interviews such as the Schedule for Affective Disorders and Schizophrenia for School Age Children (KSADS). These interviews require specific training and considerable effort. Minimally, clinicians must methodically determine the presence or absence of each *DSM* ADHD symptom and its approximate age of onset. Symptoms must be assessed in their developmental context; that is, they must be of greater frequency and severity than what is typical for others of the same sex, age, and cognitive level. Specific impairments should be documented to verify the diagnosis, establish objective treatment targets, and, if necessary justify medication use and expected duration of treatment. Most individuals with ADHD have at least one additional psychiatric disorder (see Chapters 3 and 11). Care must be taken to differentiate other disorders that might be comorbid with ADHD, as well as disorders that share ADHD features and could be misdiagnosed. The clinical evaluation should review symptoms of oppositional defiant disorder, disruptive mood dysregulation disorder, conduct disorder, anxiety, depression, mania, autism spectrum disorder, specific learning disorders, intellectual disability, substance abuse, and tic disorders.

Older individuals sometimes adapt to ADHD with lifestyle choices that minimize obvious impairments, such as choosing occupations that do not require sustained attention or denying interest in personal relationships. The clinician must assess whether these are healthy adaptations to the disorder or denial of its consequences. Given the potential for adaptation, diagnosis in adults can be based on a history of multiple impairments over the lifetime, rather than concurrent impairment in multiple domains at the time of evaluation.

Given that follow-up visits for ADHD management are often limited to brief appointments, it is crucial during the initial evaluation to consider the patient's full psychosocial context. This allows proper consideration of external factors that might affect behavior and helps identify the full range of psychosocial problems that might require intervention. In younger patients, it is necessary to assess whether one or two parents are involved, the nature of the relationship between parents, style of parenting and discipline, living arrangements, the degree to which nonparental adults participate in supervision, and nonacademic activities that the child enjoys. In older patients, it is helpful to understand living arrangements, the nature of personal support networks, and recreational interests.

Patients might or might not exhibit overactivity in the office setting. If observed, it helps corroborate ADHD, but its absence does not contradict the diagnosis. Clinicians should also be mindful that some, particularly younger, patients can be shy in unfamiliar settings, and that failures to engage with the examiner might not represent usual behavior.

Developmental Considerations in the Clinical Interview

Strategies for assessing ADHD were developed primarily from experience with school-age children. With increased awareness that ADHD occurs in all age groups, modifications in standard approaches to assessment can better address developmental differences that occur across the life span.

Preschool-Age Children

Normally high levels of distractibility and overactivity confound differentiating preschool-age children with and without ADHD. It remains unclear whether teacher-completed rating scales are as well validated and sensitive in differentiating normal and abnormal levels of hyperactivity in very young children compared to older youth. In *DSM* field trials, most patients with ADHD had greater than expected levels of hyperactivity and impulsivity by about age 4.[1] The majority of children brought for ADHD evaluations are in kindergarten or early grade school. However, increasing numbers of preschool-age children are being diagnosed and subsequently treated with medication. Difficulties that frequently occur with ADHD in this age group include sleep irregularities, excessively oppositional and defiant behavior, temper tantrums, aggression, and increased risk for accidental injuries and conflict both in and outside of the home. Preschool-age children with more severe ADHD tend to retain their diagnosis over time, although current presentations seen at initial diagnosis often change at subsequent assessments. Clinicians should also assess potential autism spectrum disorders and intellectual disabilities, as well as problems with hearing, speech and language, elimination disorders, family approaches to parenting, and overall psychosocial history.

School-Age Children

It is useful in assessing a school-age child to determine what is known or expected about the clinic visit. A question like "What did your mom tell you about why you are coming to the doctor today?" can provide a good sense of the child's insight into his or her difficulties. Diagnosis in this age group chiefly relies on parent and teacher reports. Younger children very rarely endorse ADHD symptoms or related problems. Nonetheless, it is important to include the child in the assessment, both to aid in evaluation and set the stage for treatment adherence. Direct observation might reveal obvious problems with hyperactive-impulsive behavior, although ADHD symptoms are often not evident in tightly controlled settings. If feasible, observing the child in a group setting, such as the lobby waiting area or an actual classroom, provides more valuable information about potential ADHD behaviors. Common comorbid disorders include learning disorders, autism spectrum disorders, oppositional defiant disorder, anxiety, and tic disorders.

It is reassuring when parent and teacher reports report similar patterns of ADHD symptoms. At times, clinicians will have to make sense of conflicting information. Parents and teachers might have their own biases that interfere with accurate reporting. Parental biases might reflect their own psychopathology, including depression or personal histories of ADHD, their ability to tolerate certain levels of behavioral disruption, and cultural attitudes. One parent might spend more time with the child and be a more accurate informant than the other. Parents who have ADHD themselves might be eager to intervene or might resist seeing anything wrong. Some parents are particularly motivated to obtain medication and/or academic accommodations, while others are strongly opposed to medication or are concerned about stigma if teachers and others find out about the diagnosis.

Teacher reports might also suffer from bias. Some teachers are strong proponents of ADHD, with expectations that prescription medication will help both the child and classroom management. Others resist the diagnosis, sometimes based on negative views of medication or an unwillingness to provide accommodations or special treatment for the student. Some teachers do not have time or are unwilling to complete ratings. Teachers are generally better observers of hyperactive-impulsive symptoms than inattention or distractibility.

Impairment in younger patients is generally reflected at home, school, and with peers. Since diagnosis requires evidence of symptoms and impairment in multiple settings, it is necessary to consider other sources of information if parent and teacher reports conflict. Reviewing several years' school records is very helpful. While teachers rarely make overtly critical comments on report cards, difficulties are sometimes subtly evidenced by less-than-glowing behavioral assessments. It is generally advisable to heed teacher complaints of ADHD-like difficulties when parents fail to see problems, appreciating all the potential issues of bias in parental reports. In contrast, high levels of parental complaints in the absence of any school-related difficulty suggests that family issues may be of greater concern and emphasizes the importance of a thorough psychosocial assessment.

Adolescents

Adolescents evaluated for ADHD are often either highly motivated and hoping to improve their academic performance in anticipation of college or having very severe academic, social, or family difficulties with a high risk for significant life failures. An essential goal of the initial assessment is developing a degree of trust between the adolescent patient and clinician, which is essential in subsequently developing an effective treatment strategy. It is generally advisable to begin the assessment by interviewing the adolescent alone, prior to meeting with parents, to assess the patient's motivation and goals, discuss confidentiality and its limits, and give the patient the first opportunity to describe what is going on. Good initial questions are "What is your understanding about what this meeting is for today?" or "How can I help you?" After providing the adolescent with the initial opportunity to discuss pertinent information, parents can be invited to join the session and asked to provide a long-term perspective and other missing information. It is not advisable to meet with parents without the teenager present, unless parents convey that there is highly sensitive information that they would otherwise not discuss. A teenager's normal strivings to become independent from parents, particularly regarding peer relationships, sometimes adds to family tension. At times, parents need assistance differentiating problems related to ADHD from those of normal adolescent development.

Adolescents are typically the best informants on their own current ADHD symptoms.[2] Parents can usually describe symptom patterns that began early in childhood, but they generally do not spend enough time with their teenage children to give accurate descriptions of current behavior. Teacher ratings are less valuable once students leave elementary school, as students rotate through different classrooms over the course of the day. Review of past and current academic records can provide important corroborating evidence for the diagnosis, which is particularly helpful if the patient is uncooperative.

Adolescents with ADHD often have fewer hyperactive-impulsive symptoms than younger children (see Chapter 5). Some symptoms manifest differently. For example, adolescents might complain of inner restlessness instead of overactivity. Inattention might manifest as problems with motivation, organization, and completing tasks. Failing to turn in completed assignments is a common cause of low grades. Neuropsychological testing can be particularly useful in differentiating mild or predominately inattentive ADHD from other learning disabilities.

Adolescents with ADHD are at greater risk for early initiation of nicotine use, illicit drug use, alcohol, and sexual activity, as well traffic violations and motor vehicle accidents (see Chapter 3). These risks should be assessed during the evaluation, and opportunities taken, when indicated, to provide counseling toward reducing them.

Adults

Adults generally come for evaluation from a sense of personal frustration and lack of accomplishment or due to the insistence of third parties such as spouses, partners, parents, or employers. It can be helpful to begin the interview by asking, "Why are you coming now for an evaluation of ADHD?" The questions that best identify adults with ADHD are "Are you easily distracted by extraneous stimuli?" and "If you are interrupted while doing something, is it hard to get back to what you were doing before the interruption?" Adults without clinical disorders will rarely answer yes to these questions. Positive responses are highly indicative of ADHD or another psychiatric disorder.

Adult patients are generally the primary informants in their own evaluations. Parents, spouses, partners, and others, if available, can provide useful corroborating information, but their involvement is limited due to privacy needs. *DSM* criteria require some evidence of symptoms before age 12.

Adults with superior cognitive abilities or strong levels of academic support might experience their symptoms and related impairment until they face demands of higher education, full-time employment, or living independently. Problems with inattention and executive function often have greater relevance for adults. Common difficulties include problems related to organization, distractibility, time management, and following through on important tasks. Psychiatric comorbidity is the rule and not the exception. Common comorbid conditions include lifetime histories of conduct disorder or antisocial behavior, nicotine dependence, other substance abuse or dependence, depression, anxiety disorders, and risky behaviors (see Chapters 3 and 11).

Some clinicians remain skeptical of the validity of adult ADHD and continue to view adults seeking evaluations as primarily malingering or drug seeking. Reliance on adult self-report of ADHD symptoms appears as a major concern, although doubts about symptom self-report do not generally extend to the diagnosis of other psychiatric disorders. Corroboration of self-reported history of ADHD symptoms with past records, third-party reports, and an overall life course consistent with the known developmental outcomes of the disorder remain the best approach to establishing an ADHD diagnosis.

Medical Assessment

Patients diagnosed by nonmedical clinicians require medical assessment prior to initiation of medication. Physicians, regardless of specialty, should conduct a medical assessment as part of their evaluation. This includes review of current and significant past illnesses, surgeries, current and past chronic medication history, major accidents and physical injuries, and possible loss of consciousness. Specialist physicians should confirm that the patient has had necessary primary care and health maintenance, including appropriate physical examinations and immunizations. If appropriate for the patient's developmental level, the potential onset of risky behaviors, such as nicotine, drug, and alcohol use, motor vehicle use, and sexual activities, should be discussed. The clinical interview provides an additional opportunity to counsel patients on reducing these risks, such as the use of seat belts, not drinking and driving, and safe sex practices.

Some general medical conditions can mimic or cause ADHD symptoms and should be considered in the context of other history. Obstructive sleep apnea or other sleep disorders, seizure disorders, and endocrine disorders, such as thyroid disease and diabetes, should be considered in the context of other supportive history.

Physical examination is not typically necessary if the patient has received appropriate general medical management. Measuring height, weight, and vital signs is the standard of care. Height and weight should always be documented in children and adolescents. Blood pressure should be documented for older patients. If abnormal motor movements or vocalizations, that is, tics, are present, their nature, frequency, and intensity should be documented. Vision and hearing tests are not standard but might be considered if indicated by specific history.

Screening for Cardiac Risk

Due to baseline rates of sudden death among individuals under age 35, it is necessary to screen for cardiac risk prior to initiation of ADHD pharmacotherapy. Key questions should be asked of all patients (Box 6.1) and answers recorded. These are the same questions that are assessed in youth sports physicals. A positive response to any of these suggests the need for further cardiac evaluation prior to medication treatment. In the absence of positive responses, it is generally accepted that additional cardiac workup is unnecessary. The American Heart Association supports obtaining electrocardiograms (EKGs) if one is deemed necessary, but routine EKG screening is not generally indicated or considered useful (see Chapter 12).

Family History

Given the high heritability of ADHD, it is not uncommon to identify other family members with or likely to have the disorder. The evaluation should review the family history for other evidence of learning and academic difficulties, mood and anxiety disorders, and problems with substance abuse and/or antisocial behavior. While positive family history does not confirm an ADHD diagnosis, the information is helpful in corroborating the diagnostic picture. It can also prove useful in treatment planning, particularly if one or both parents are also affected.

Educational Testing

Approximately half of individuals with ADHD have other measurable learning impairments. Some assessment for learning disability should be part of any

---

Box 6.1 Screening Questions for Identification of Potential Cardiac Risk Factors for Sudden Death

Is there any history of:
    Unexplained shortness of breath with exercise?
    History of poor exercise tolerance?
    Fainting or seizures with exercise?
    Palpitations with exercise?
    Family history of sudden or unexplained death in first- or second-degree relatives?
    Long QT syndrome or other hereditary arrhythmias?
    Wolff-Parkinson-White syndrome?
    Cardiomyopathy, heart transplant, pulmonary hypertension, or an implantable defibrillator?
    Hypertension?
    Organic (not functional) heart murmur?
    Other cardiac abnormalities?

Answering "yes" to any question should prompt review by an appropriate specialist in cardiology prior to initiation of medication.

Source: Adapted from Warren et al.[4]

Box 6.2 Tests to Assess Learning Disabilities

Tests of Intellectual Function

Wechsler Preschool and Primary Scale of Intelligence (WPPSI)	Preschool age
Wechsler Intelligence Scale for Children (WISC)	School age
Wechsler Adult Intelligence Scale (WAIS)	Adults

Tests of Adaptive Functioning or Developmental Level

Denver Developmental Screening Test	Preschool age
Vineland Scales of Adaptive Behavior	

Tests of Academic Achievement

Woodcock Johnson Tests of Achievement
Wechsler Individual Achievement Test (WIAT)
Wide Range Achievement Test (WRAT)
Nelson-Denny Reading Test

ADHD evaluation. Appropriate tests provide estimates of intellectual ability and academic achievement, as well as adaptive functioning, if there are questions of intellectual disability (Box 6.2). Learning disabilities are diagnosed when discrepancies exist between measured intellectual level and academic achievement. Screening tests can be sufficient for an initial assessment with an option to follow up with more comprehensive testing if specific difficulties are suspected.

Some practical considerations, such as cost and access to testing, impede routine screening for learning disabilities in ADHD evaluations. Physicians do not typically perform these examinations, which necessitates referral to a psychologist or educational specialist. Private medical insurance companies rarely cover the expense of educational testing, asserting that schools are obligated to assess learning disabilities. Schools themselves have limited resources and can resist or delay evaluations. Clinicians can gain a broad sense of whether testing is necessary by reviewing academic records and standardized tests scores. Any student who consistently underperforms in school or scores below average on standardized testing should be screened specifically for learning disabilities. Families can be advised to self-pay for testing if they have adequate financial resources. Alternatively, parents can be encouraged to demand assessments from their school districts. This is generally initiated by submitting a written request to the school's guidance office.

Non-Evidence-Based Approaches to Assessment

There is great public interest in assessing ADHD with approaches that are less subjective than clinical interviews and appear to be based on more objective scientific measures. Many clinicians utilize these methods, possibly to improve their own perception of diagnostic certainty, create a veneer of science-based practice, or increase revenue. Although several of these have revealed interesting research findings, their diagnostic specificity in those investigations is always based on gold-standard clinical interviews. Routine clinical use of these approaches adds considerable expense to health care costs and has not, as yet, provided added patient benefit.

Neuropsychological Testing

Some clinicians administer larger batteries of neuropsychological tests to assess ADHD. Neuropsychological testing has proven useful in identifying underlying patterns of cognitive difficulties in ADHD, particularly in areas of attention control and executive functioning. However, these deficits are identified in only about half of patients with ADHD, and there is no correlation between cognitive findings and *DSM* symptoms. Neurocognitive findings provide no information that is predictive of long-term outcome or treatment response. There is no proven benefit for the routine use of extensive neuropsychological testing in evaluating ADHD per se.

Computerized Tests of Attention

Commercially available computerized tests of attention, such as the Test of Variable Attention (TOVA) or the Conners' Continuous Performance Test (CPT), have appeal as objective laboratory measures. These tests can be administered in the clinician's office in about 20 minutes. Patients respond to different stimuli by pushing a button. This records errors of commission (i.e., pushing the button in the absence of a proper stimulus) and omission (i.e., failing to push the button when required), as well as an estimate of reaction time. Results are compared to known profiles of people with and without ADHD. Clinicians are able to charge for the tests as diagnostic procedures.

The main limitation of these tests is that results are neither sensitive nor specific for the diagnosis. Many patients with ADHD excel at computer games and do not show predicted deficits. Numerous psychiatric and neurological conditions are associated with deficits in attention and response inhibition. Despite their potential appeal, computerized tests of attention have no added value for assessing ADHD.

Electroencephalography

Some research suggests that patients with ADHD exhibit different patterns of brain electrical activity as measured by EEG, particularly increased theta power.[3] While these findings provide a basis for future research on ADHD neurobiology, EEG results have poor predictive power for the diagnosis itself. Obtaining an EEG is clinically indicated only in the context of history or physical findings suggestive of seizures or other neurological disorders as evidenced by functional deterioration or specific neurological symptoms.

Brain Imaging Studies

There is great interest in using brain imaging modalities for ADHD diagnosis. Considerable research has consistently shown differences in brain structure, function, and developmental trajectories in groups with and without ADHD (see Chapter 4). However, it is essential to recognize that these studies assess group effects, and there is a great deal of variability among individuals within each group. No data suggest that brain imaging findings for individual patients have predictive power for the diagnosis. Some practitioners represent that they can diagnose ADHD and other psychiatric conditions on the basis of neuroimaging, particularly using single-photon emission tomography (SPECT) and positron emission tomography (PET) imaging. There are no scientific data to support this, and patients and families do not appreciate that the radiation risk of these procedures is not outweighed by any potential benefit.

Laboratory Studies

There is no role for other laboratory studies, specifically blood and urine tests, in routine assessment of ADHD. On rare occasions, clinical histories might suggest an indication for specific tests. Testing for serum lead is reasonable with a suspicion of lead toxicity because of where the child lives or with a history of pica. Endocrine studies, such as thyroid tests and fasting blood glucose, might be indicated if clinical symptoms suggest possible endocrine disorders. Urine and blood toxicology screens are useful with clinical suspicion of illicit drug use. Although much research has demonstrated genetic contributions to ADHD risk, none of these findings is specific to the disorder and there is no justification for genetic testing as an assessment tool.

References

1. Lahey BB, Applegate B, McBurnett K, et al. DSM-IV field trials for attention deficit hyperactivity disorder in children and adolescents. *Am J Psychiatry*. 1994;151:1673–1685.

2. Wilens T, McBurnett K, Bukstein O, et al. Multisite controlled study of OROS methylphenidate in the treatment of adolescents with attention-deficit/hyperactivity disorder. *Arch Pediatr Adolesc Med*. 2006;160:82–90.

3. Loo SK, Makeig S. Clinical utility of EEG in attention-deficit/hyperactivity disorder: a research update. *Neurotherapuetics*. 2012;9:569–587.

4. Warren AE, Hamilton RM, Bélanger SA, et al. Cardiac risk assessment before the use of stimulant medications in children and youth: a joint position statement by the Canadian Paediatric Society, Canadian Cardiovascular Society, and the Canadian Academy of Child and Adolescent Psychiatry. *Can J Cardiol*. 2009;25;625–630.

Further Reading

Kooij SJ, Bejerot S, Blackwell A, et al. European consensus statement on diagnosing and treatment of adult ADHD: The European Network Adult ADHD. *BMC Psychiatry*. 2010;67.

Nass RD. Evaluation and assessment issues in the diagnosis of attention deficit hyperactivity disorder. *Semin Pediatr Neurol*. 2006;12:200–216.

Chapter 7

Treatment Planning

Children and Adolescents

> ## Key Points
>
> - Multimodal approaches to ADHD treatment in youth have proven successful in maximizing improved global functioning.
> - Pharmacotherapy is the only intervention to yield large treatment effects on core ADHD symptoms.
> - Optimal ADHD management usually combines medication treatment with psychosocial interventions that target patient-specific difficulties.

ADHD medications were first introduced with the caveat that they be used only when psychosocial and behavioral therapies had proven inadequate. As the pervasive consequences of ADHD became evident, a view developed that multimodal approaches to treatment, that is, medication management combined with a comprehensive range of psychosocial interventions, were optimal for behavioral improvement and long-term outcomes. This strategy was tested in the landmark Multimodal Treatment Study of ADHD (MTA), which randomized children to 14 months of intensive medication management, intensive behavioral therapy, combination medication and behavioral therapy, or community-based treatment.[1] While the study demonstrated that medication management was most effective for acute control of ADHD symptoms, combination medication and behavioral interventions yielded the best improvement in overall functioning. The general approach to treatment of ADHD in youth since the MTA Study has been an emphasis on pharmacotherapy combined with specific psychosocial treatments matched to individual patient needs.

Treatment usually requires a team approach that coordinates various interventions in office, family, and school settings. This includes services by physicians, psychologists, teachers, and other mental or behavioral health professionals. Optimal integration of these services can vary based on the background and strengths of the lead clinician, as well as family needs and resources. Psychiatrists, pediatricians, other primary care specialists, psychologists, and other mental health experts likely differ in expertise as well as the time they have available for clinic visits. A critical component of successful treatment planning rests on the ability of the lead clinician to provide necessary care or appropriate referral to collaborating clinicians who can assist in patient management. This approach is consistent with the medical home model developed by the American Academy of Pediatrics.

Assessment

More time is typically available for initial assessments than for follow-up visits. During the initial evaluation, clinicians optimally obtain a comprehensive view of ADHD symptoms and impairments within the context of the patient's family and social functioning (see Chapter 6). It is easier to assist with subsequent difficulties if the full range of patient problems is identified at the start of treatment. The initial assessment also establishes a level of rapport between the clinician and family, which can facilitate long-term treatment adherence and success.

Major areas of concern for children and adolescents with ADHD are difficulties that impact life at home, school, and with peers. Assessing the degree to which an individual has problems within these domains is the first step in developing a comprehensive treatment plan. Standard approaches to ADHD treatment target single or multiple domains, and they include family, academic, social, and individual interventions (Fig. 7.1).

Once a diagnosis is made, clinicians should provide feedback that summarizes the diagnostic impression and places the patient's difficulties in context with what is known about ADHD. Patients and families often find reassurance in learning that their problems are not unique but fall into patterns that are similar to others with the disorder. It is also useful to describe aspects in which the individual patient is unique. This provides a solid basis for discussion of appropriate treatment options.

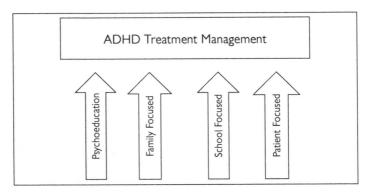

Figure 7.1 Multimodal approaches to ADHD treatment.

Psychoeducation

Psychoeducation provides information about ADHD that goes beyond diagnostic feedback and discussion of treatment options.[2] Psychoeducation should begin once the diagnosis is given and should continue throughout clinical care. Psychoeducation is an accepted evidence-based treatment for several adult psychiatric disorders, including schizophrenia and bipolar disorder. Similarly, it is shown to be useful in managing ADHD, a disorder with potential lifelong consequences requiring ongoing patient involvement to optimize treatment adherence.

Psychoeducation ideally presents didactic information about ADHD, its consequences, and strategies for intervention. There are numerous approaches to incorporating psychoeducation into an ADHD management plan. Useful formats include informal discussion, structured lectures, slides and videos, provision of brochures and information sheets, or referral to books, websites, and support groups (Box 7.1). Skill development through role-play and problem-solving exercises has proven useful. Psychoeducation is appropriate for parents and children with ADHD. Its emphasis properly shifts to patient education during adolescence when teenagers are inclined to assume more responsibility for personal decision making. Psychoeducation is also useful for teachers and other professionals who interact with ADHD-affected youth.

Psychoeducation can be incorporated into regular medication visits, behavioral therapies, family counseling sessions, and professional development programs. It can be structured into single didactic sessions or comprehensive workshops. Outcome studies indicate that psychoeducational programs increase parent and teacher awareness, improve maternal well-being and competence, increase patient and family satisfaction, decrease social stigma among patients and other family members, decrease family conflict, and improve compliance with prescribed medication regimens.[2]

Family-Focused Interventions

It is naïve to assume that pharmacotherapy is sufficient to control all ADHD-related impairments. Family interventions can play a primary role with very young children, in patients with milder ADHD, when medications are ineffective or not tolerated, or when parents are strongly opposed to medication use.[3] Family treatments are particularly useful with comorbid oppositional defiant disorder or anxiety. Combination approaches result in greater parent satisfaction than medication alone.

With abuse, significant family chaos, economic hardship, marital difficulties, or other severe stressors, environmental influences are likely to overwhelm any benefit derived from medication and attempts at effective parenting. Clinicians must remain cognizant of broader social factors, which are likely to require interventions that go beyond standard approaches to ADHD.

ADHD

Box 7.1 Resources for Families

Support Groups

Attention Deficit Disorder Association (ADDA)
www.add.org
Children and Adults with Attention Deficit Disorders (CHADD)
www.chadd.org
Edge Foundation
www.edgefoundation.org
Learning Disabilities Association of America (LDA)
www.ldanatl.org

Informative Websites

American Academy of Child and Adolescent Psychiatry (AACAP):
Facts for Families
http://www.aacap.org/AACAP/Families_and_Youth/Facts_for_
Families/Facts_for_Families_Pages/Children_who_Cant_Pay_Attention_
ADHD_06.aspx.
Healthy Children
http://www.healthychildren.org/English/health-issues/conditions/adhd/
Pages/Understanding-ADHD.aspx?
National Institute of Mental Health (NIMH)
http://www.nimh.nih.gov/health/publications/adhd/
complete-publication.shtml
US Centers for Disease Control and Prevention
http://www.cdc.gov/ncbddd/adhd/

Books

Barkley RA. *Taking Charge of ADHD, Third Edition: The Complete Authoritative Guide for Parents.* Guilford Press; 2013.
Monastra VJ. *Parenting Children With ADHD: 10 Lessons That Medicine Cannot Teach.* American Psychological Association (APA); 2005.
Pope L, Oswald HM. *Colleges That Change Lives: 40 Schools That Will Change the Way You Think About Colleges.* Penguin Books; 2012.
Wilens TE. *Straight Talk About Psychiatric Medications for Kids, Third Edition.* Guilford Press; 2008.

Behavioral Parent Training

Children and adolescents with ADHD are often difficult to manage and contribute to significant stress within families and between parents. This situation can be worsened if one or both parents have ADHD. In typical situations, successful approaches to parenting ADHD-affected children are similar to those that are useful in parenting most children.

Behavioral parent training methods used in the MTA Study are widely available, easy to implement, and associated with positive overall improvements in child behaviors.[4] Behavioral improvements are not specific to core ADHD symptoms. Training also contributes to increased parent confidence and reduced parent stress.

Social learning theory suggests that antecedents and consequences largely drive behavior, and that parents can modify their children's behaviors by changing their own approach to parent–child interactions. Parent training programs primarily aim to teach parents implementation of behavioral and cognitive techniques proven useful in modifying problematic childhood behaviors. Programs designed specifically for parents of children with ADHD also commonly add a psychoeducational component on the nature and consequences of the disorder.[3]

Parent training is suitable for individual or group settings.[5] The overarching goal is to improve positive interaction patterns between parents and children and decrease parents' coercive and negative responses to unwanted behaviors. More specific goals include recognizing the importance of structure and consistency, reducing harsh and critical parenting, and avoiding discipline approaches that are either lax or overly punitive. Other common topics include improving child management by setting consistent limits and expectations, increasing use of positive attention to increase appropriate behaviors, and developing a set of responses to negative behaviors that includes ignoring, time-out, and natural consequences.

Programs are typically organized into 1- to 2-hour weekly sessions conducted over 10 to 20 weeks.[5] Sessions can be structured so that participants learn and master one skill before progressing to the next. Participants learn to identify common parenting errors by watching recorded vignettes, generate solutions and alternatives based on their understanding of behavioral techniques, and practice appropriate parenting skills with role play. Homework between sessions reinforces key concepts from the lesson. Specific skills often include design and implementation of daily "report card" and associated reward systems for home behaviors; focusing on praise, reward, and positive reinforcement; how to ignore minor annoyances and undesired behaviors; how to give effective commands; establishing "when-then" contingencies and the importance of warnings and transitions; and the appropriate use of "time-out."

It is useful for clinicians to approach parents of younger children as co-therapists whose role is to modify behaviors at home through the application of appropriate behavioral techniques. As older children and adolescents gain the cognitive capacity to understand the consequences of their actions, behavioral interventions shift to the larger family and include efforts to improve communication, problem solving, limit setting, and behavioral contracting to agree on expected parental responses to positive and negative child behaviors.

Several programs similar to behavioral parent training are designed specifically for preschool-age children.[6] Parent Child Interaction Training (PCIT) attempts to improve parent–child interactions using two basic interventions. First, in child-directed interaction, parents engage their child in play to improve their general relationship. Second, in parent-directed interaction, parents learn specific behavioral management skills as they play with their child. Another form of parent training is the Community Parent Education Program (COPE), which also focuses on improving parent–child relationships and development of more effective parent management skills. Each of these, PCIT and COPE, is an evidence-based intervention with strong empirical support.

Other Family Therapies

Other types of family therapy might be appropriate for specific circumstances. For example, marital or relationship therapy might improve severe parental discord; bereavement therapy or grief counseling might be appropriate following a death or other loss; family therapy might be indicated in following trauma or abuse. Proper management of parental ADHD can be essential to optimize overall family functioning (see Chapter 8).

School-Focused Interventions

Proper classroom placement and educational planning are essential components of ADHD management.[7] School interventions for ADHD differ from those designed to address specific learning disabilities. Families and schools vary on the level of resources they can provide for school-based ADHD treatment. Given those limitations, students should be placed in optimal academic environments with appropriate educational services.

Schools receiving US federal dollars are legally required to meet the educational needs of all students. Success in fulfilling this mandate is dependent in part on local school standards and budgetary constraints. It is sometimes helpful for families to obtain educational advocates or other legal aid to assist in obtaining necessary services. While some private schools emphasize programs designed for students with ADHD and other behavioral or learning difficulties, they have no legal obligation to provide special services.

Section 504 Plans

Section 504 plans are required by the Federal Rehabilitation Act of 1973 to ensure that students with disabilities attending elementary and secondary schools receive appropriate modifications in educational services to support their academic success and access to learning. Section 504 plans can be implemented in regular classrooms, regular classrooms with supplemental pullouts for resource assistance, or in specialized, self-contained classrooms. Typical academic modifications provided under these plans include preferential classroom seating, extended time on tests, taking examinations in less distracting areas, breaks during examinations, and modified or reduced homework assignments. These modifications have little financial cost, but successful implementation depends on cooperation from the classroom teacher.

Students are eligible for 504 plans if they have a physical or mental impairment that limits a major life activity, such as attending school. Schools establish specific procedures and criteria to determine eligibility under federal guidelines. A clinician's note attesting to an ADHD diagnosis is generally not sufficient to obtain services. Clinicians should direct parents to request evaluations for 504 plans through the child's school counseling office. A multidisciplinary committee determines eligibility based on information derived from an array of sources, including medical records, psychoeducational tests, teacher recommendations, social and cultural factors, and physical limitations. Schools are obligated to conduct their own evaluations, but they may consider outside testing reports if available. Parents have the right to appeal though a due process hearing if they disagree with the committee's assessment and recommendations.

Individualized Educational Programs

An individualized educational program (IEP) is required by the Federal Individuals With Disability Education Act (IDEA) to ensure that students with disabilities who attend elementary and secondary schools receive specialized instruction and related services necessary for their educational success. Services under IEPs go beyond 504 plans and can include time and resources for academic tutoring, provision of 1:1 classroom aides, placement in self-contained special education classrooms, additional individual or group counseling, placement in a publically funded private school, or other services. Eligibility procedures are similar to 504 plans.

Behavioral Classroom Management

Behavioral classroom management uses approaches that are similar to behavioral parent training and can be particularly effective when implemented in conjunction with behavioral approaches used at home.[4] Implementation of behavioral classroom management depends on the classroom teacher and incorporates contingency management procedures that include daily report cards, point systems and reward programs, and appropriate use of time-out. This approach is the basis for specialized school programs for ADHD, but some teachers implement them for individual students in regular classrooms. Behavioral classroom management results in moderate treatment effects on disruptive behavior, attention to instruction, rule compliance, and work productivity.

Standardized Testing Accommodations

Schools may allow students to take extra breaks during examinations and also provide a quiet environment to take tests. Students with ADHD and additional learning disabilities can sometimes obtain untimed or extended time on standardized tests and college entrance examinations. These modifications can be extremely helpful when students are otherwise qualified academically, but limited in their performance by ADHD. Criteria and procedures for obtaining extended examination time are typically listed on the testing organizations' websites. As with 504 plans and IEPs, eligibility usually requires some level of psychoeducational testing that goes beyond certification of a clinical diagnosis.

Patient-Focused Interventions

Health Maintenance

Regardless of who coordinates ADHD treatment, all patients ideally have a primary care physician to oversee general health maintenance. This includes periodic physical examinations, charting growth trajectories, and timely administration of recommended immunizations. Co-occurring general medical conditions, such as dermatological, endocrine, or neurological disorders, should be managed appropriately in conjunction with ADHD therapy.

Health maintenance as a specific focus of ADHD management can be organized with a developmental focus. With younger children, clinicians should counsel parents on maintaining safety within and outside the home, including use of bicycle and skateboard helmets and wearing seat belts while driving. With older youth, clinicians should address safety issues pertaining to high-risk activities frequently seen in adolescents with ADHD, including recreational drug and alcohol use, sexual activity, and reckless driving.

Pharmacotherapy

Pharmacotherapy is likely to be recommended for most patients (see Chapter 10). Selection of a particular ADHD medication can depend on prior response or nonresponse, family preference, ease of administration, required duration of effect, tolerability, presence of comorbidities, and other factors. An initial titration period is generally advised before a specific medication and optimal dose can be prescribed. Clinicians should present medication as part of an integrated treatment strategy and not as the sole solution to a patient's difficulties.

Social and Peer-Related Activities

Children and adolescents with ADHD demonstrate a range of social competence. Some are popular and talented, despite other difficulties. Others, particularly those with autism spectrum disorder, have substantial peer-related problems. As children progress through elementary and middle school, social interactions are increasingly important in shaping self-perception, interests, and preferred activities. Promotion of positive peer skills and social relationships is a critical component of ADHD treatment.

Children sometimes develop a negative sense of themselves because they take medication or attend therapy. The optimal way to improve social interactions is by supporting a child's ability to be successful in typical, age-appropriate activities with friends and peers. To the extent that they are able, parents should actively facilitate play dates and other peer interactions. Parents should also encourage participation in activities in which their child expresses interest and can develop a level of competence and enjoyment. Examples include team or individual sports, music, art, drama, or other structured activities typically enjoyed at a given age.

Social Skills Training

Some children are unable to develop appropriate peer interactions with simple participation in age-appropriate activities. Social skills training programs help develop and improve individual social skills.[4] These programs follow models similar to those used in behavioral parent and classroom management training. Group social skills sessions can be conducted weekly, often in conjunction with psychoeducation or parent management training for adults. Specific goals of social skills programs include helping participants to modify verbal and nonverbal behaviors so they can be more successful in social situations. As with parent training programs, videos, role play, and homework are used to reinforce learning specific social skills. Lessons might address learning to wait your turn, calling someone on the telephone, inviting yourself into a playgroup, recognizing emotions in others, and generating alternatives to deal with frustration and disappointment. Social skills programs have been implemented in clinics, schools, summer camp programs, and other venues. Currently, available research evidence neither supports nor refutes the potential value of social skills training as a component of ADHD treatment.[8]

Individual Psychotherapy

Individual psychotherapy, including cognitive-behavioral therapy, has not proved useful in pediatric ADHD and is rarely recommended in this age group. Appropriate forms of individual psychotherapy might be useful and considered for difficulties often associated with ADHD, such as anxiety, depression, or low self-esteem.

Promoting Treatment Adherence

Psychosocial and behavioral ADHD treatments are usually time limited. Medication therapy requires long-term use for ongoing response. Follow-up studies up to 5 years demonstrate sustained clinical benefit with ongoing medication use. Nonetheless, despite this and the immediate apparent effects of most ADHD medications, one quarter to one third of patients obtain only one prescription and one half to two thirds discontinue treatment within 1 year. Similar to many chronic medical conditions, promoting long-term adherence to ADHD treatment remains a challenge.

Numerous factors improve long-term adherence.[9] Most important is maintenance of an ongoing clinician–patient relationship. Patients are more likely to remain in treatment after more thorough initial evaluations; if they understand ADHD as a neurodevelopmental disorder; if they undergo initial short-term titration with low, medium, and high medication doses; and if they have frequent monitoring visits with dose adjustments to optimize benefits and decrease side effects. Current Federal DEA regulations require clinical assessment prior to medication renewal no less frequently than every 90 days. Insisting that patients come for clinic visits at least once every 3 months, and generally refusing to approve refills outside of clinic visits, complies with federal laws and promotes better treatment compliance. Adherence is improved further when insurance is available to cover costs, when once-daily medication formulations are used, and when there is a lack of social stigma among family and peers regarding medication use.

Younger children typically comply with their prescribed medications when given to them by parents. For older children and adolescents, acceptance of medication is more likely when the patient has been involved in treatment decision making and when there is clear evidence of benefit. Authoritarian demands on older youth are rarely successful in changing behaviors. Instead, motivational interview techniques can guide older patients toward recognizing how medication is useful in helping them accomplish their own goals. For example, a teenager might be willing to take medication on schooldays if he or she wishes to attend a good college but might refuse medication on weekends because of side effects. Accepting the patient's input into the treatment plan is likely to be more beneficial than rigidly insisting that medication must be taken without question.

References

1. The MTA Cooperative Group. A 14-month randomized clinical trial of treatment strategies for attention-deficit/hyperactivity disorder. *Arch Gen Psychiatry.* 1999;56:1073–1086.

2. Montoya A, Colom F, Ferrin M. Is psychoeducation for parents and teacher of children with ADHD efficacious? A systematic literature review. *European Psychiatry.* 2011;26:166–175.

3. Zwi M, Jones H, Thorgaard C, York A, Dennis JA. Parent training interventions for attention deficit hyperactivity disorder (ADHD) in children aged 5 to 18 years. *Cochrane Database Syst Rev.* 2011;12:CD003018.

4. Pelham WE, Fabiano GA. Evidence-based psychosocial treatments for attention-deficit/hyperactivity disorder. *J Clin Child Adolesc Psychol.* 2008;37:184–214.

5. Forehand R, Jones DJ, Parent J. Behavioral parenting interventions for disruptive behaviors and anxiety: what's different and what's the same? *Clin Psychol Rev.* 2013;33:133–145.

6. Charach A, Carson P, Fox S, Ali MU, Beckett J, Lim CG. Interventions for preschool children at high risk for ADHD: a comparative effectiveness. *Pediatrics* 2013;131:e1584–1604.

7. Semrud-Clikeman M, Bledsoe J. Updates on attention-deficit/hyperactivity disorder and learning disorders. *Curr Psychiatry Rep.* 2011;13:364–373.

8. Storebo OJ, Skoog M, Damm D, Thomsen PH, Simonsen E, Gluud C. Social skills training for attention deficit hyperactivity disorder (ADHD) in children aged 5 to 18 years. *Cochrane Database Syst Rev.* 2011;12:CD008223.

9. Charach A, Fernandez R. Enhancing ADHD medication adherence: challenges and opportunities. *Curr Psychiatry Rep.* 2013;15:371–379.

Further Reading

Fiks AG, Mayne S, Debartolo E, Powers TJ, Guevara JP. Parental preferences and goals regarding ADHD treatment. *Pediatrics.* 2013;132:692–702.

Subcommittee on Attention-Deficit/Hyperactivity Disorder, Steering Committee on Quality Improvement and Management. ADHD: clinical practice guidelines for the diagnosis, evaluation, and treatment of attention- deficit/hyperactivity disorder in children and adolescents. *Pediatrics.* 2011;128:1007–1022.

Chapter 8

Treatment Planning

Adults

Key Points

- There is a substantial evidence base supporting pharmacotherapy for adult ADHD.
- Preliminary evidence supports a potential role for psychosocial interventions, including psychoeducation, cognitive behavioral and other therapies, school and workplace accommodations, coaching, and support groups.
- Optimal treatment generally combines medication management with problem-specific interventions selected for individual patients.

For most emotional and behavioral disorders, pediatric treatment strategies are generally derived from those developed initially in adults. ADHD is one disorder in which management of adults is guided by well-established approaches to treating children. Pharmacotherapy remains the only adult treatment with well-established evidence based on large controlled studies. However, pharmacotherapy is rarely sufficient to address the full range of adult impairments. Research on adult multimodal interventions is increasing, but development of adult psychosocial and behavioral therapies lags far behind established approaches for children. The challenge with adults is to integrate medication use with problem-specific psychosocial interventions that are most likely to optimize functioning in individual patients. Comprehensive treatment planning for adults might include psychoeducation, medication management, individual or group therapies, coaching, school or work accommodations, advocacy, and support groups (Table 8.1).[1] The most useful interventions tend to be brief, well-structured, skill-oriented, and specific to ADHD.

Assessment

Treatment planning begins with the initial assessment (see Chapter 6). Given that more time is generally allotted for evaluation compared with follow-up visits, the initial appointment provides a unique opportunity to establish the diagnosis, assess potential comorbidities, identify current symptoms, and quantify

Table 8.1 Treatment Modalities for Adult ADHD

Multiple Positive Controlled Trials	Single Randomized or Large Uncontrolled Trials	Expert Opinion, Open Studies, and Anecdotal Reports
Stimulant medications	Cognitive-behavioral therapies	Academic accommodations
Nonstimulant medications		Adaptive technology
		Advocacy groups
		Coaching
		Couples therapy
		Educational planning
		Occupational accommodations
		Psychoeducation
		Support groups
		Vocational counseling

specific treatment targets. Optimally, the clinician obtains sufficient information about the individual's life to understand the full psychosocial context of ADHD-related difficulties. At assessment's end, the clinician should provide diagnostic feedback and specifically convey an integrated view of how ADHD has affected the person. Improved long-term treatment adherence is associated with more comprehensive initial assessments, increased patient self-awareness, and patient participation in choosing initial management options.[2]

Unlike children who rarely have insight into the nature and consequences of the disorder, many adults recognize a link between ADHD symptoms and lifetime difficulties. Children often have little motivation for treatment, and implementation of psychosocial interventions is largely dependent on parent and teacher efforts. In contrast, successful adult treatment depends almost entirely on the patient's motivation and commitment. Recognition in the initial assessment of an individual's readiness to change provides a framework for subsequent treatment planning.

Psychoeducation

Psychoeducation should begin in tandem with the initial assessment and continue throughout treatment.[3] Individuals who are well informed about ADHD and how it affects them are more likely to contribute to treatment planning decisions and remain adherent over time. Ideally, psychoeducation should include the patient, spouse or partner, and possibly other family members. Useful topics address ADHD symptoms and typical impairments, prevalence rates, the natural course of the disorder, common comorbidities and associated risks, heritability, neurobiology, and management approaches.

An improved understanding of ADHD and its related effects can assist patients in recognizing that their problems are not unique but are understandable in the context of a well-recognized disorder. Psychoeducation reduces stigma and can decrease hostility among other family members as they gain greater understanding of ADHD and its consequences. Integration of psychoeducation into the overall management plan enhances the relationship between patient and clinician and is associated with increased long-term treatment success.

Health Maintenance

Ideally, patients have primary care physicians who manage general medical health needs. Unfortunately, many adults with ADHD fail to obtain adequate medical care. Physicians who prescribe ADHD medications should be mindful of their patients' general medical status and refer to appropriate providers as needed. Patient weight and vital signs should be monitored routinely. Chronic medical conditions, such as endocrine disorders or hypertension, should be appropriately controlled.

Adults with ADHD often make lifestyle choices that are inconsistent with good health maintenance (see Chapter 3). When indicated, ADHD treatment provides an opportunity for counseling on diet, weight control, smoking, drug and alcohol use, and risky behaviors such as driving and sexual activity. Physicians managing ADHD should assume a broader medical role than simply writing prescriptions.

Medication Management

Treatment algorithms for medication selection in adults are less established than those for younger patients (see Chapters 10 and 11). The FDA has approved both stimulant and nonstimulant ADHD medications for adults. As with children, adult clinical trials consistently show larger treatment effect sizes for stimulants versus nonstimulants (Fig. 8.1).[4] Potential benefits of any stimulant are easily assessed with short-term titration. Larger effect sizes, safety, and ease of titration support the recommendation to use stimulants as first-line adult treatments, similar to pediatric ADHD. Atomoxetine is also indicated for adults and provides a second-line alternative if stimulants prove unsatisfactory.

Some clinicians have ongoing concerns about stimulants, drug misuse, and illicit diversion (see Chapter 12). Studies suggest that the risk of abuse, that is, using medication to get high or for recreational purposes, is small, particularly with some extended-release formulations. Clinicians should counsel older adolescents and adults not to sell or share their medication with others. Clinicians are obligated to maintain careful medication records, including dates, strengths, and quantities prescribed. Any patterns of lost prescriptions or seeking additional prescriptions should be noted and addressed appropriately with the patient. Nonstimulants might be appropriate first-line treatments in patients with histories of serious substance use difficulties or other medication misuse.

ADHD medications are largely formulated to meet the needs of children who attend school and have after-school homework and activities.

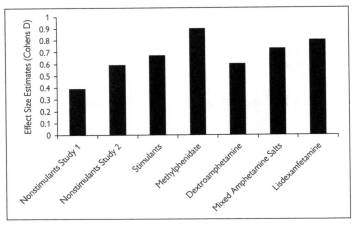

Figure 8.1 Estimated medication effect sizes for adult ADHD. (Adapted from Moriyama et al.[4])

Many adults have work schedules or other obligations that exceed the 8- to 12-hour duration of effect that is usually provided by a single dose of an extended-release stimulant. Some adults require medication for most of their waking hours, while others need benefits only while at work or school. A review of the patient's schedule and related needs should inform the clinician's recommendations on choice of a specific medication and dosing regimen. With stimulants, an initial titration should assess response on various doses of a single-daily dose extended-release formulation (see Chapter 10). Once the optimal medication and dose are determined, complementary doses of the same medication in an immediate-release form can extend the duration of treatment effect. Some nonstimulants, notably atomoxetine, have associated improvements up to 24 hours after dosing, which is potentially useful when medication is required throughout waking hours. Unlike stimulants, nonstimulants must be taken daily to maintain effects. Clinicians should not prescribe nonstimulants to patients who will not agree to take the medication daily.

Educational Planning and Academic Accommodations

Older adolescents and young adults should develop educational plans that promote individual interests, strengths, and long-term objectives.[1] Attending a traditional 4-year college might or might not be the best choice for someone with ADHD. Reasonable plans might include attendance at a junior college or trade school, joining the military, or beginning to work. For those attending college, acknowledging one's ADHD and associated limitations, as well as utilizing available resources, can aid in accomplishing academic goals.

Students attending postsecondary schools should contact their institution's office of disability services and consider requesting educational accommodations. Although potential long-term benefits of accommodations have not been systematically studied, anecdotal evidence suggests they are useful.[5] Typical accommodations include provision of note-taking services and books on tape, extended test time, taking tests in distraction-free examination areas, alternative forms of examinations, substitutions for required courses, modified assignments, academic tutoring, and priority in course registration. In some cases, testing agencies provide modifications for postgraduate entrance examinations such as the MCAT or LSAT, as well as for state and national licensing examinations.

Student disability offices and test-specific websites provide recommendations on current requirements for accommodations. Accommodations are granted based on legal requirements to assist individuals with disabilities that substantially interfere with major life functions. To protect against students faking symptoms, multiple sources of information, including medical and academic records, third-party observations, and neuropsychological tests should be considered during assessment (see Chapter 12).[5] Documenting ADHD alone is insufficient. Eligibility requires clearly demonstrating that ADHD symptoms contribute to substantial impairments in academic activities. Assessments must be recent and reflect current functioning.

There is ongoing controversy as to whether impairment should be established relative to an individual's measured aptitude, others with whom the student competes academically, or the general population.[5] In the United States, courts have ruled in favor of both the educational-peer and general population standard for modifications on high-stakes standardized tests. Nonetheless, there is a growing trend to use the general population standard. This can make it extremely difficult to obtain accommodations for graduate or professional school entrance or licensing examinations.

Vocational Counseling and Work Accommodations

Assisting adults in finding suitable occupations is a critical component of treatment planning.[1] Adults with ADHD often have occupational difficulties due to poor matching between job requirements and their own strengths and limitations. Some adults with ADHD are very successful when self-employed or with jobs that provide flexible work schedules, physical activity, or high levels of stimulation. Vocational testing and counseling can be useful for those with uncertain occupational interests and objectives.

Under the Americans With Disabilities Act, employees are entitled to reasonable accommodations at work for disabilities that "substantially limit a major life activity." Companies with 15 or more employees are obligated to provide accommodations under the Act. As with academic accommodations, eligibility requires clear documentation of the diagnosis and related impairments. Employees wishing to obtain accommodations must disclose their diagnosis and apply in writing to their supervisor or company's human resources department. The employee must be otherwise qualified for the position and requested accommodations cannot create an undue employer burden. Typical accommodations include working in distraction-free areas, flexible scheduling to allow work during periods of higher productivity, working at home, assigning work that better utilizes an employee's strengths and minimizes the need for weaker skills, and providing assistance devices or software that supports efforts at organization and effective time management.

Individual Therapies

Medications are at best estimated to reduce ADHD symptoms by 50%, leaving patients with significant residual difficulties. For some, individual therapy potentially provides further improvement. Several ADHD-specific forms of individual therapy have preliminary evidence of treatment effectiveness. These are increasingly available in community settings and should be considered for appropriate patients.

Cognitive-Behavioral Therapy

Cognitive-behavioral therapy (CBT) appears to be ineffective for pediatric ADHD. Unlike children and adolescents, adults seeking treatment generally have greater awareness of their deficits and are motivated to improve. Early studies, including some controlled trials, suggest that CBT is effective for adults, particularly in conjunction with adequate medication management.[6] The theoretical basis for CBT rests on the assumption that core ADHD symptoms arise from underlying deficits in sustained attention, inhibitory control, working memory, and motivation. These lead to lifetime underachievement, contributing to false and negative beliefs that reinforce ongoing dysfunction and limit development of adequate coping skills.

Successful CBT programs are time limited, requiring an average of 10 sessions, and are highly structured. Programs typically teach ADHD-specific compensatory skills and include opportunities to practice between sessions, usually in conjunction with a workbook. Programs address both emotional and cognitive strategies. Emotional strategies seek improvements in emotional regulation, impulse control, motivation, and self-esteem. Cognitive strategies emphasize learning to recognize mental distortions, setting priorities, improved organization and planning, problem solving, anger and stress management, relationship issues, mindfulness, and psychoeducation. Interventions address maladaptive thought patterns that limit acquisition of adaptive life skills. Behavioral skills are overpracticed until they are automatic, contributing to overall functional improvement. Therapist manuals and patient workbooks organized into individual training modules and based on effective CBT programs have been published and are commercially available (Box 8.1).

ADHD Coaching

ADHD coaching is increasingly popular, although research supporting its effectiveness is limited.[7] Coaching has potential value for individuals having particular difficulties with motivation, time management, and organization. Coaching attempts to change life skills directly, often using motivation and reward.

> **Box 8.1 Resources for Adult ADHD Cognitive-Behavioral Therapy Programs**
>
> **For Patients and Families**
> Safren SA, Sprich S, Perlman CA, Otto MW. *Mastering Your Adult ADHD: A Cognitive-Behavioral Treatment Program Client Workbook (Treatments That Work)*. Oxford University Press; 2005.
>
> **For Clinicians**
> Safren SA, Perlman CA, Sprich S, Otto MW. *Mastering Your Adult ADHD: A Cognitive-Behavioral Treatment Program Therapist Guide (Treatments That Work)*. Oxford University Press; 2005.
>
> Solanto MV. *Cognitive-Behavioral Therapy for Adult ADHD: Targeting Executive Dysfunction*. Guilford Press; 2011.

Coaching is similar to CBT in that its emphasis is behavioral and not insight oriented. Unlike CBT, which focuses on general approaches and skills likely to be useful in a variety of contexts, coaching is primarily directed toward specific goals and objectives. While CBT is usually conducted in time-limited, formally structured sessions, coaches are generally available as needed and sessions tend to be flexible, brief, and frequent. Coaches work in individual or group settings and might utilize phone, text, and e-mail messages to prompt adaptive behavior. Standards and core competencies for coaching have been established, although coaches are generally unlicensed and have a variety of educational backgrounds.

Other Individual Psychotherapies

Other forms of psychotherapy are appropriately recommended depending on individual needs. Problems related to anxiety or depression, substance abuse, relationship difficulties, or self-esteem are all potential indications for psychotherapy. These therapies are generally not specific for ADHD but address problems that commonly co-occur with the disorder.

Marital and Couples Therapy

Adults with significant marital or relationship difficulties might benefit from couples therapy. Couples therapy promotes a realistic joint understanding of ADHD, its effects on the relationship, and potential changes in the relationship for mutual benefit.[1] It is also critical to avoid blaming the ADHD-affected individual or the disorder for all of the couple's difficulties. Similarly, it is important to avoid using an ADHD diagnosis as an excuse for inconsiderate or irresponsible behavior.

Group Therapies

Group interventions are a time and cost-effective means of providing helpful care. There has been considerable interest in developing group treatments for adult ADHD, and some have shown preliminary effectiveness in small controlled trials. Group therapies typically empha-size methods to improve attention and acquisition of compensatory skills for disorder-related deficits. Group treatments also provide support for individual participants.

Dialectical Behavioral Therapy Groups

Dialectical behavioral therapy (DBT) groups were originally developed for treatment of borderline personality disorder. Although borderline person-ality disorder and ADHD are distinct, they share common difficulties with emotional regulation, impulse control, low self-esteem, and interpersonal relationships. There is some initial success using DBT groups for ADHD.[8] Treatment is organized into time-limited weekly sessions. Specific modules address psychoeducation, mindfulness training, dysfunctional behavior analy-sis, emotion regulation, impulse control, depression, organization strategies, relationships, stress management, and substance abuse. In preliminary trials, treatment effects on ADHD symptoms were small but significant, with larger improvements seen with general health and mood. DBT might play an adjunc-tive role with ADHD medication, particularly in adults with overreactivity and other mood symptoms.

Metacognitive Therapy

Group metacognitive therapy is a manualized treatment developed for ADHD that provides CBT with a particular focus on time management, organization, and planning.[8] The program is highly structured and organized into weekly sessions that emphasize making new skills automatic through repeated practice. One initial open pilot study demonstrated significant improvements in medicated individuals on measures of attention and execu-tive function.

Cognitive-Behaviorally Oriented Group Rehabilitation

Cognitive-behaviorally oriented group rehabilitation also uses a CBT approach to address ADHD symptoms and related difficulties.[8] Treatment occurs in 10 to 12 weekly sessions that are organized around review of previous home-work, introduction of a new topic, new homework, and a self-reflective assessment of the day's program. Topics typically address ADHD neurobiol-ogy and pharmacotherapy, motivation and activity initiation, communication, impulse control, managing comorbidity, and self-esteem. An initial open pilot demonstrated improvements in ADHD and related mood symptoms.

Use of Technology and Devices

Although their use has not been assessed scientifically, many clinicians encourage patients to make full use of new technologies to aid in ADHD management.[1] Apps and other programs for smart phones, tablets, and other devices are increasingly available to help manage time and organize contacts, schedules, and assignments. Mobile devices can be programmed to provide alarms and reminders for certain tasks. Automatic payment plans are easily established and ensure that individuals pay bills promptly.

Advocacy and Support Groups

Some adults wish to participate in support or advocacy groups. Among others, patients and families can be referred to two national organizations, Children and Adults With Attention Deficit Disorders (CHADD) (www.chadd.org) and the Attention Deficit Disorder Association (ADDA) (www.add.org). Each sponsors annual national meetings as well as many local chapters and regional events. Group websites are excellent sources of current information.

References

1. Murphy K. Psychosocial treatments for ADHD in teens and adults: a practice-friendly review. *J Clin Psychol.* 2005;61:607–619.

2. Charach A, Fernandez R. Enhancing ADHD medication adherence: challenges and opportunities. *Curr Psychiatry Rep.* 2013;15:371–379.

3. Kooij SJ, Bejerot S. Blackwell A, et al. European consensus statement on diagnosis and treatment of adult ADHD: The European Network Adult ADHD. *BMC Psychiatry.* 2010;10:67.

4. Moriyama TS, Polanczyk GV, Terzi FS, Faria KM, Rohde LA. Psychopharmacology and psychotherapy for the treatment of adults with ADHD—a systematic review of available meta-analyses. *CNS Spectrums.* 2013;6:1–12.

5. Weyandt LL, DuPaul GJ. ADHD in college students: developmental findings. *Dev Dis Res Rev.* 2008;14:311–319.

6. Mongia M, Hechtman L. Cognitive behavioral therapy for adults with attention-deficit/hyperactivity disorder: a review or recent randomized controlled trials. *Curr Psychiatry Rep.* 2012;14:562–567.

7. Kubik JA. Efficacy of ADHD coaching for adults with ADHD. *J Atten Disord.* 2010;13:442–453.

8. Knouse LE, Cooper-Vince C, Sprich S, Saffren SA. Recent developments in the psychosocial treatment of adult ADHD. *Expert Rev Neurother.* 2008;8:1537–1548.

Further Reading

Harrison AG, Rosenblum Y. ADHD documentation for students receiving accommodations at the postsecondary level. *Can Fam Physician.* 2010;56:761–765.

Manos MJ. Psychosocial therapy for adults with attention-deficit/hyperactivity disorder. *Postgrad Med.* 2013;125:51–64.

Murphy K, Ratey N, Maynard S, Sussman S, Wright SD. Coaching for ADHD. *J Atten Disord.* 2010;13:546–552.

Rostain AL, Ramsay JR. A combined treatment approach for adults with ADHD—results of an open study. *J Atten Disord.* 2006;10;150–159.

Chapter 9

Basic Pharmacology

Key Points

- Approved ADHD medications include stimulants and nonstimulants.
- ADHD medications influence catecholamine activity in the prefrontal cortex (PFC) and to varying degrees enhance ratios of preferred "signal" to nonpreferred "noise" pathways, leading to improved attention and motor control.
- The PFC functions optimally within a narrow range of catecholamine activity, but dose effects of ADHD medications vary widely.
- Extended-release stimulant formulations are designed to maximize the duration of ascending pharmacokinetic profiles and avoid potential tolerance to steady-state or decreasing plasma drug concentrations.

Since Bradley's discovery in the 1930s that amphetamine (AMPH) improved concentration and behavior in hyperactive children, medication has been the mainstay of ADHD treatment (see Chapter 2). Virtually all psychotropic drugs have been considered as potential ADHD pharmacotherapies. Those proven effective generally enhance central noradrenergic and dopaminergic signaling, or increase noradrenergic activity alone.

The Universe of ADHD Medications

The ADHD medication armamentarium includes agents with Food and Drug Administration (FDA) or other regulatory agency approval, as well as drugs used off-label (Table 9.1). Stimulants are regarded as most effective with the most robust treatment effect sizes.[1] FDA-approved nonstimulants are atomoxetine, a noradrenergic reuptake inhibitor, and the alpha-2 agonists, guanfacine extended-release (ER) and clonidine ER. Commercially available medications prescribed off-label include immediate-release (IR) alpha-2 agonists, certain wake-promoting agents, tricyclic and some other antidepressants, antipsychotic agents, and monoamine oxidase inhibitors.

Stimulants

Stimulants have been proven safe and efficacious in over 300 controlled clinical studies.[2] It is commonly stated that 70% of patients respond favorably

Table 9.1 The Universe of ADHD Medications

FDA-Approved Medications		Off-Label Medications
Stimulants	**Nonstimulants**	
		Immediate-release alpha-2 agonists
Methylphenidates	Atomoxetine	Buproprion
D-Methylphenidates	Extended-release alpha-2 agonists	Modafinil
D-Amphetamines		Tricyclic antidepressants
Mixed amphetamine salts		Antipsychotics
Lisdexamfetamine		Monoamine oxidase inhibitors

to stimulants. In fact, approximately 70% respond favorably to the first stimulant prescribed, whether a methylphenidate (MPH) or amphetamine (AMPH).[3] Of those who fail, an additional 70% respond favorably to the alternative class. As such, more than 90% of patients have satisfactory clinical improvement with stimulants, at least during acute treatment. Some patients respond preferentially to one or another stimulant class, but there is no method other than clinical trial and error to predict whether MPH or AMPH is the optimal choice.

Stimulants are typically effective within an hour of dosing, but symptoms return once medication wears off. Ongoing use is necessary to maintain improvement. All have similar potential side effects. The most common is appetite loss, which is highly dose dependent. Other common side effects include weight loss, sleep disturbance, nausea, abdominal pain, headache, dizziness, dry mouth, and dysphoria (see Chapter 10). Some of these are seen frequently in patients taking placebo and might be associated with ADHD itself and not medication.[4] Increased irritability or "rebound hyperactivity" can occur when drug effects wear off in late afternoon (see Chapter 10). There is clear evidence that ADHD medications, particularly stimulants, can decelerate growth, particularly during the first 18 months of therapy (see Chapter 12). All MPH and AMPH formulations are Schedule II drugs, suggesting a high risk for abuse, and require use of controlled prescriptions in many jurisdictions. A black box warning informs on potential abuse. There are class warnings on cardiovascular risks.

Methylphenidates

A summary of MPH formulations appears in Table 9.2. Immediate-release MPH (MPH-IR, Ritalin®, Methylin™), more specifically d,l-MPH, contains a 50/50 racemic mixture of *d-threo* and *l-threo* isomers. MPH has been used since the 1960s, when it was viewed as milder and less prone to abuse than AMPH. Prior to introduction of effective ER stimulant formulations, MPH-IR accounted for more than 90% of ADHD prescriptions. A single isomer IR formulation, *d-threo*-MPH (d-MPH-IR, Focalin®), was introduced in 2001. Both MPH-IR and d-MPH-IR typically have effect onsets within 30

Table 9.2 FDA-Approved Methylphenidate (MPH) Formulations for ADHD

Brand Name	Doses Available	Usual Dosing*
Immediate Release (MPH-IR)		
Ritalin®	2.5, 5, 10, 20 mg	5 mg–20 mg/bid–tid; Max 60 mg/day:
Methylin™	2.5, 5, 10 mg chew 10 mg/5 ml solution	Children: 2.5–10 mg/bid–tid Adults: 5–15 mg/bid–tid
Focalin®	2.5, 5, 10 mg	2.5–10 mg/bid; max 20 mg/day
Sustained Release (MPH-SR)		
Ritalin SR®	20 mg	20–60 mg/qd–bid Max 60 mg/day
Metadate ER®	20 mg	20 mg–60 mg/qd–bid Max 60 mg/day
Extended Release (MPH-ER)		
Concerta®	18, 27, 36, 54 mg	Children: 18–54 mg/day Adults: 18–72 mg/day
Ritalin LA®	10, 20, 30, 40 mg	Children: 20–40 mg/day Adults: 20–60 mg/day
Metadate CD®	10, 20, 30, 40, 50, 60 mg	20–60 mg/day
Daytrana®	10, 15, 20, 30 mg patch	10–30 mg/day; 9 hours wear
Quillivant XR™	25 mg/5 ml solution	20–60 mg/day
Focalin XR®	5, 10, 15, 20, 25, 30, 35, 40 mg	Children: 10–30 mg/day Adults: 10–40 mg/day

*May exceed FDA dosing.

bid, twice daily; qd, once daily; tid, three times daily.

to 45 minutes after administration, are effective for approximately 4 to 6 hours, and require 2 or 3 times daily dosing to maintain improvements into early evening.[5] Regular tablets cannot be crushed, but chewable tablets (Methylin™) and liquid (Methylin™ solution) are options if swallowing pills is difficult.

Sustained-release preparations (MPH-SR, Ritalin-SR®, Metadate-ER®) were introduced to avoid lunchtime dosing while maintaining symptom control over an 8-hour school day.[5] These formulations embed MPH in a waxy matrix that dissolves after ingestion and gradually releases medication over time. Although popular among some, little evidence suggests that MPH-SR has longer effect durations than MPH-IR. SR formulations are increasingly dispensed as generic equivalents of brand name MPH-ER, but they fail to provide equal benefits.

Beginning in the late 1990s, several technologies allowed creation of MPH-ER formulations that are effective 8 to 12 hours after dosing.[5,6] The

OROS (Osmotic [Controlled] Release Oral [Delivery] System) formulation (OROS-MPH, Concerta®) is a multicompartment capsule comprising MPH, osmotic control agents, and a rate-controlling membrane. Once ingested, a capsule overcoat immediately releases MPH similar to MPH-IR. As the capsule proceeds through the gut, fluids enter the OROS chamber and force medication out through a laser-drilled hole, leading to an ascending plasma profile similar to MPH-IR administered three times daily at 4-hour intervals. The capsule must be swallowed intact, and it cannot be crushed, divided, chewed, or dissolved in liquid. OROS-MPH has been shown in classroom laboratory studies to be effective for 10–12 hours, although shorter durations are sometimes reported in clinical settings.

Several MPH-ER formulations (Ritalin LA®, Metadate CD®, Focalin XR®) use pulsed-release beaded technologies and combine mixtures of immediate and delayed-release MPH or d-MPH.[5,6] IR beads enter circulation rapidly and initiate medication effects. Delayed-release beads are initially protected with a coating that dissolves after exposure to intestinal fluids to release a second bolus of MPH or d-MPH approximately 4 hours after ingestion. Improvement can persist 8 to 12 hours. For patients unable to swallow pills, these formulations can be opened and sprinkled on food.

Two additional MPH-ER compounds are particularly useful when swallowing is difficult. The MPH transdermal system (MTS, Daytrana®) is a drug-containing patch that is applied each morning and worn 9 hours under clothing. One unique feature is enhanced control of treatment onset and offset. Since the patch creates an MPH reservoir in the skin, benefits persist for up to 3 hours after patch removal.[1] Although MTS is appealing for younger children who resist swallowing, one major impediment is frequent development of skin irritation under the application site. A liquid MPH-ER (Quillivant XR™) is also available, and classroom laboratory studies suggest up to 12 hours of improvement compared with placebo.

Amphetamines

Racemic dl-AMPH was synthesized in the late 1880s and eventually marketed in aerosol form as a bronchodilator. Various AMPH formulations have been used for ADHD, beginning with Bradley's initial use of dl-AMPH (Benzedrine) in 1937 (see Chapter 2). Concerns in the 1960s and 1970s over AMPH abuse risks led to a preference for MPH in ADHD treatment, although few data exist to confirm differences between the two. A summary of AMPH formulations appears in Table 9.3.

Immediate-release d-AMPH (d-AMPH-IR, Dexedrine®, Dextrostat®) is generally effective within an hour of administration.[5] D-AMPH-IR typically remains effective 4 to 6 hours after ingestion and requires dosing 2 or 3 times daily to maintain daylong benefit. A second IR-AMPH formulation, mixed amphetamine salts (MAS-IR, Adderall®), contains equal parts dl-AMPH aspartate monohydrate, d-AMPH saccharate, d-AMPH sulfate, and dl-AMPH sulfate, providing a 3:1 ration of d- to l-AMPH. MAS-IR was originally marketed as the weight loss medication Obitrol®. However, amphetamines are no longer indicated for weigh loss due to risks of abuse. Similar to d-AMPH-IR, MAS-IR generally reduces ADHD symptoms for 4–6 hours and requires multiple daily dosing to maintain improvements.

Table 9.3 FDA-Approved Amphetamine (AMPH) Formulations for ADHD

Brand Name	Doses Available	Usual Dosing*
Immediate Release (AMPH-IR)		
Dexedrine® Dextrostat®	5, 7.5, 10, 15, 20, 30 mg	2.5–40 mg/qd–tid Max 40 mg/day
Adderall®	5, 7.5, 10, 12.5, 15, 20, 30 mg	5–40 mg/qd–tid Max 40 mg/day
Vyvanse ®	20, 30, 40, 50, 60, 70 mg	30–70 mg/day
Sustained Release (AMPH-SR)		
Dexedrine® spansules®	5, 10, 15 mg	5–40 mg/qd–bid Max 60 mg/day
Extended Release (AMPH-ER)		
Adderall XR®	5, 10, 15, 20, 30 mg	Children: 5–30 mg/day Adults: 5–60 mg/day

*May exceed FDA dosing.

bid, twice daily; qd, once daily; tid, three times daily.

Sustained-release d-AMPH (d-AMPH-SR, Dexedrine® Spansule®, Dexedrine® SR) contains two forms of beads with half released immediately and the remainder released gradually over several hours. However, no differences were found in studies comparing duration effects of d-AMPH-IR and d-AMPH-SR. AMPH-SR formulations remain available but are rarely used.

An ER preparation of mixed AMPH salts (MAS-ER, Adderall XR®) uses a two-phased pulsed-released formulation to deliver 50% of MAS beads immediately, followed by a second pulse approximately 4 hours later.[5,6] In laboratory studies, MAS-ER provided significant benefits compared to placebo up to 12 hours after dosing. Clinically, most patients improve for 8–12 hours. Capsules can be opened and sprinkled on food if swallowing is difficult.

Lisdexamfetamine (LDX, Vyvanse®) is an AMPH prodrug formed by covalent bonding of d-AMPH with the amino acid lysine. LDX is a prodrug and not psychoactive as the parent compound. Once ingested and absorbed, LDX is cleaved through enzymatic processes located on red blood cells into separate lysine and d-AMPH molecules. Since enzymatic hydrolysis of AMPH occurs slowly, the delayed release reduces the abuse risks seen with other stimulants that can be inhaled or injected to provide rapid euphoria and cocaine-like effects. LDX is available in 20, 30, 40 50, 60, and 70 mg capsules, which can be opened and mixed with water if a patient has difficulty swallowing without affecting the slow-release properties. Total AMPH released in 30, 50, and 70 mg LDX is roughly equivalent to 10, 20, and 30 mg of MAS-XR, respectively. Classroom laboratory studies have shown positive differences on ADHD symptoms between LDX and placebo for up to 14 hours after dosing, although shorter effect durations can be seen in clinical settings.[1]

Nonstimulants

Several FDA-approved nonstimulants are summarized in Table 9.4. Given lower response rates and smaller treatment effect sizes, nonstimulants are regarded as second-line medications.[2,5] They are particularly useful when stimulants are ineffective or not tolerated, concerned about high risk for stimulant misuse, addressing certain comorbid conditions, and in combination with stimulants to improve tolerability or enhance treatment response.

Atomoxetine

Atomoxetine (Strattera®) is a noradrenergic reuptake inhibitor. The medication is available in capsule form and cannot be opened or sprinkled. Atomoxetine is primarily metabolized by CYP2D6 hepatic enzymes, which creates the potential for interactions with many other drugs and increased toxicity in slow metabolizers. Dosing is weight based. The recommended dose range is 1.2–1.4 mg/kg per day up to 100 mg. The maximum dose of 1.8 mg/kg per day was established as a safety threshold for patients who might be CYP2D6 slow metabolizers. Concomitant administration with fluoxetine or other medications that inhibit CYP2D6 will cause the patient to become a slow atomoxetine metabolizer with increased risk for elevated plasma concentrations and concomitant adverse events.

Atomoxetine is useful when stimulants are not tolerated, particularly when irritability is a stimulant side effect, or when comorbid tic or anxiety disorders are present. Atomoxetine has a mild beneficial effect on tic expression and has proven efficacy as a single agent for both ADHD and comorbid anxiety symptoms. When effective, atomoxetine lacks the daily on/off effects seen with stimulants and has been shown to decrease ADHD symptoms at least 24 hours after dosing. Also unlike stimulants, benefits appear to increase with sustained use, with maximal treatment effects 3–4 weeks after initiating the full dose. However, if no response is in evidence after 1 week of the maximum dose, it

Table 9.4 FDA-Approved Nonstimulant Medications for ADHD		
Brand Name	**Doses Available**	**Usual Dosing**
Noradrenergic Reuptake Inhibitors		
Strattera® (atomoxetine)	10, 18, 25, 40, 60, 80, 100 mg	Begin 0.5 mg/kg per day Increase to 1.2–1.4 mg/kg per day Max 100 mg/day Give qd or divided bid
Alpha-2 Agonists		
Intuniv® (guanfacine-ER)	1, 2, 3, 4 mg	1–4 mg/qd*
Kapvay® (clonidine-ER)	0.1, 0.2 mg	0.1–0.4 mg/day, qd or divided bid*

*Pediatric dosing only. Not approved for adult use.

bid, twice daily; ER, extended release; qd, once daily.

is unlikely that subsequent benefits will be seen. Atomoxetine can be administered as a single daily dose or divided twice daily in morning and evening. Twice daily dosing decreases side effect risk and enhances 24-hour responses. Since symptom reductions are dependent on sustained use, patients who frequently miss prescribed doses are likely to lose treatment benefit.

The side effect profile differs from stimulants. Common side effects include headache, nausea, and drowsiness. These often subside after initial titration. Atomoxetine is usually initiated at approximately 0.5 mg/kg per day to reduce side effect risk. Doses are best increased at no less than weekly intervals until the optimal target dose is reached.

Alpha-2 Agonists

Alpha-2 agonists were originally approved as antihypertensive agents, but they are effective for ADHD.[2,5] Two ER formulations, guanfacine-ER (Intuniv®) and clonidine-ER (Kapvay®), have FDA approval for ADHD in pediatric age groups, both as monotherapies and in combination with stimulants. Patients require blood pressure monitoring, particularly when treatment is initiated. For either agent, clinicians should begin with the lowest dose and increase by the smallest available increment, as tolerated, but no more frequently than once weekly. Somnolence is often the limiting factor during dose titration, but it generally improves over time. Other common side effects include headache, abdominal pain, disrupted sleep, fatigue, and dizziness. Guanfacine-ER is given once daily, either in morning or at night. Clonidine-ER can be administered once or twice daily.

Interestingly, although alpha-2 agonists are sedating, their primary benefit in ADHD appears to be on inattentive symptoms.[7] Some evidence suggests that combination alpha-2 agonist and stimulant treatment enhances cognition and leads to greater ADHD improvement than with either monotherapy. Alpha-2 agonists suppress tics and are particularly useful, alone or in stimulant combination, in treating ADHD with comorbid tic disorders.

Off-Label Medications

IR guanfacine (Tenex®) and clonidine (Catapres®) are commonly used in off-label ADHD treatment, either as monotherapy or in combination with a stimulant.[2,5] Guanfacine is available in 1 and 2 mg tablets and usually administered in 0.5 to 1.5 mg doses given twice daily. Clonidine is available in 0.1, 0.2, and 0.3 mg tablets and usually administered in.05 to.1 mg doses given one to three times daily. Other off-label therapies are typically employed only when FDA-approved medications are proven unsatisfactory. These include the wake-promoting agent modafinil; tricyclic antidepressants; buproprion; venlafaxine; the antipsychotics haloperidol, risperidone, and aripiprazole; and monoamine oxidase inhibitors. Most of these have limited evidence of benefit and/or associated safety concerns that necessitate special monitoring.

Drug Targets and Mechanisms of Action

Most ADHD medications act directly in the central nervous system to increase synaptic levels of the catecholamines dopamine and/or norepinephrine (Fig. 9.1).[8] Increased norepinephrine activity appears essential for symptom reduction, but optimal ADHD treatment seems to require perturbation of both noradrenergic and dopaminergic systems. AMPH has a broader range of drug targets than MPH. Both AMPH and MPH inhibit catecholamine reuptake into presynaptic neurons by blocking norepinephrine and dopamine transporters. AMPH further directly displaces norepinephrine and dopamine from presynaptic storage vesicles, and it inhibits monoamine oxidase and subsequent neurotransmitter breakdown. The direct action of atomoxetine is similar to MPH, but it is selective for blockade of noradrenergic and not dopaminergic transporters.

Recent research suggests that ADHD treatment response is not a direct effect of increased catecholamine release, but that increased levels of norepinephrine and dopamine have indirect modulating effects on glutaminergic signaling in the prefrontal cortex (PFC) (Fig. 9.2).[9] PFC circuits are intrinsically involved in ADHD and regulate processes related to attention, executive function, motor inhibition, emotion regulation, and reward. One subset of PFC networks mediates active attention to "preferred" inputs or "signals," while another subset mediates attention to "nonpreferred" inputs or noise. Ion channels in neuronal membrane in preferred PFC networks are kept open by cyclic adenosine monophosphate (cAMP). Activation of alpha-2 adrenergic receptors on these neurons, directly by alpha-2 agonists or indirectly by increased norepinephrine, inhibits cAMP with subsequent ion channel closure and enhanced neuronal signaling in preferred directions. Conversely, activation of the dopamine-1 receptor by increased dopamine on nonpreferred networks increases cAMP with subsequent ion channel opening, decreased circuit connectivity, and reduced attention to noise.

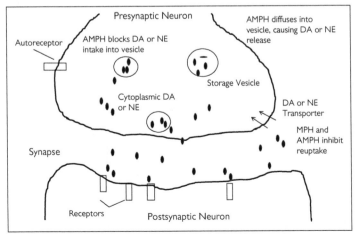

Figure 9.1 Stimulant drug targets. AMPH, amphetamine; DA, dopamine; MPH, methylphenidate; NE, norepinephrine.

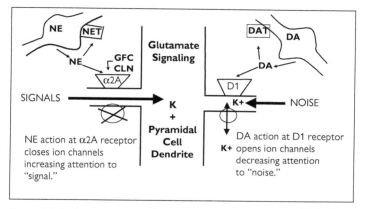

Figure 9.2 Prefrontal cortex network connections. α2A, alpha-2a receptor; D1, dopamine 1 receptor; DA, dopamine; DAT, dopamine transporter; NE, norepineph- rine; NET, norepinephrine transporter. (Adapted from Arnsten and Rubia.[9])

Stimulant Pharmacodynamics and Acute Tolerance

ADHD treatment can be viewed as a rebalancing of "signal" to "noise" ratios, either through indirect effects of increased catecholamines or direct effects of alpha-2 agonists on glutaminergic signaling in the PFC.[10] Ideally, individuals should appropriately focus on important tasks (signal), while retaining some awareness of background activity (noise) and the ability to shift attention flex- ibly when required. Optimal balancing of signal to noise ratios in the PFC is dependent on a narrow range of catecholaminergic activity. If catecholamine levels are excessively elevated, perhaps from too high medication doses or stress, PFC networks collapse with concomitant deteriorations in cogni- tion and motor control. Dopamine increases that might be useful for tasks requiring highly focused attention could also cause problems with overfocus, cognitive rigidity, and a loss of personality and spontaneity. This view is con- sistent with older work that posited separate "inverted U-shaped" stimulant dose–response curves for cognition and behavior, in which improvements increase with increasing doses up to an optimal point, followed by response deterioration.[11] Related work suggested that optimal doses for improved attention are lower than those necessary to improve behavior, suggesting that medication doses required to control overactivity might, in fact, impede cog- nitive functioning. No absolute stimulant plasma concentration predicts clini- cal improvement. Individuals with and without ADHD generally have similar cognitive and behavioral responses to stimulants, but optimal doses vary from person to person. Individual dose–response relationships likely depend on multiple factors including age, sex, and genetic polymorphisms.

Little evidence suggests that patients become tolerant to medication effects with sustained treatment (see Chapter 12). However, there has been much debate over the possibility of acute tolerance, or tachyphylaxis, with ADHD stimulants.[12] Compelling evidence, particularly with MPH, suggests that stimulant effects diminish rapidly when plasma drug concentrations are stable, and that it is important to maintain an ascending plasma drug profile to sustain symptom response.[13] This is consistent with earlier observations that strongest stimulant responses occur during the absorption phase of the plasma drug profile with maximum effects seen at the time of maximum drug concentration (Tmax). Evidence supporting the possibility of stimulant tachyphylaxis is strongest for MPH, although some research suggests it occurs with some forms of AMPH. Theories of acute tolerance explain the lack of expected efficacy in SR stimulant formulations designed to achieve steady-state plasma concentrations. Ideas about acute tolerance and the need to maintain ascending plasma concentrations are particularly relevant when choosing multiple daily stimulant doses.

Stimulant Pharmacokinetics

D-MPH-IR is readily absorbed when taken orally and reaches peak plasma levels in 1–2 hours. Its half-life (T1/2) is approximately 3–4 hours. The l-isomer has much poorer absorption, with plasma levels approximating 1% of d-MPH. MPH is primarily de-esterified to ritalinic acid via carboxylesterase 1 (CES1). A CES1 polymorphism is associated with elevated plasma MPH levels. Maximum plasma concentration (Cmax) and time to maximum concentration (Tmax) are increased when MPH is taken with food or alcohol.

D-AMPH-IR is also rapidly absorbed with a Cmax of 3–4 hours, although its T1/2 is approximately 11 hours. As with MPH, the duration response is not related to drug half-life and the largest effects occur prior to Cmax. Significant, but decreasing, effects compared against placebo continue for several hours thereafter. About half of ingested AMPH is metabolized by the liver with the remainder excreted unchanged in the urine. The major hepatic pathway is through CYPD3A4 enzymes. A genetic variant for this enzyme, more common in African Americans, leads to decreased metabolism and possible increases in Cmax. A secondary pathway is mediated by CYP2D6. CYPD2D6 polymorphisms can result in slower metabolism with possibly increased Cmax and risk of side effects. Highly acidic foods, such as grapefruit, enhance urinary excretion, leading to decreases in plasma concentration and drug half-life.

While ideas about stimulants and acute tolerance are not universally accepted, they were a guiding force for the development of virtually all currently available once-daily ER stimulants.[6] These are largely formulated to sustain the ascending plasma drug concentration and extend Tmax. AMPH formulations exhibit longer benefits beyond Tmax than MPH. Interestingly, theories of acute tolerance do not appear to apply to LDX, which reportedly demonstrates up to 14 hours of benefit with a mean Cmax of 4–5 hours.[14] LDX also exhibits less pharmacokinetic variability than equivalent doses of MAS-XR, suggesting more reliable release of active AMPH over the desired period of treatment benefit and less residual AMPH 24 hours after dosing.[14]

Pharmacokinetic profiles and potential for acute tolerance are relevant in consideration of generic stimulants. For approval of generic substitutes, the FDA requires 80% to 120% bioequivalence for Cmax and area under the plasma concentration-time curve (AUC) values compared with an approved brand-name medication. While sensible for medications with clear therapeutic windows, using this approach with ADHD stimulants does not address the critical importance of ascending plasma drug profiles on treatment response. Generic substitutes might well be less effective than branded drugs for ADHD if they lack comparable ascending drug concentration profiles.

References

1. Wigal SB. Efficacy and safety limitations of attention-deficit hyperactivity disorder pharmacotherapy in children and adults. *CNS Drugs.* 2009;23:21–31.

2. Biederman J, Spencer TJ. Psychopharmacological interventions. *Child Adolesc Psychiatr Clin N Am.* 2008;17:439–458.

3. Elia J, Borcherding BG, Rapoport JL, Keysor CS. Methylphenidate and dextroamphetamine treatment of hyperactivity: are there true nonresponders? *Psychiatry Res.* 1991;36:141–155.

4. Barkley RA, McMurray MB, Edelbrock CS, Robbins K. Side effects of methylphenidate in children with attention deficit hyperactivity disorder: a systemic, placebo-controlled evaluation. *Pediatrics.* 1990;86:184–192.

5. Daughton JM, Kratochvil CJ. Review of ADHD pharmacotherapies: advantages, disadvantages, and clinical pearls. *J Am Acad Child Adolesc Psychiatry.* 2009;48:240–248.

6. Connor DF, Steingard RJ. New formulations of stimulants for attention-deficit hyperactivity disorder. *CNS Drugs.* 2004;18:1011–1030.

7. Sallee F, Connor DF, Newcorn JH. A review of the rationale and clinical utilization of α2-adrenoceptor agonists for the treatment of attention-deficit/hyperactivity disorder. *J Child Adolesc Psychopharmacol.* 2013;23:308–319.

8. Arnsten SF, Pliszka SR. Catecholamine influences on prefrontal cortex function: relevance to treatment of attention deficit hyperactivity disorder and related disorders. *Pharmacol Biochem Behav.* 2011;99:211–216.

9. Arnsten AF, Rubia K. Neurobiological circuits regulating attention, cognitive control, motivation, and emotion: disruptions in neurodevelopmental disorders. *J Am Acad Child Adolesc Psychiatry.* 2012;51:356–367.

10. Gamo NJ, Wang M, Arnsten AF. Methylphenidate and atomoxetine enhance prefrontal function through α2-adrenergic and dopamine D1 receptors. *J Am Acad Child Adolesc Psychiatry.* 2010;49:1011–1023.

11. Swanson J, Baler D, Volkow ND. Understanding the effects of stimulant medication on cognition in individuals with attention-deficit/hyperactivity disorder: a decade of progress. *Neuropsychopharm Rev.* 2011;36:207–226.

12. Swanson J, Gupta S, Guinta D, et al. Acute tolerance to methylphenidate in the treatment of attention deficit hyperactivity disorder in children. *Clin Pharmacol Ther.* 1999;56:1073–1086.

13. Swanson J, Gupta S, Lam A. et al. Development of a new once-day formulation of methylphenidate for the treatment of attention-deficit/hyperactivity disorder. *Arch Gen Psychiatry.* 2003;60;204–211.

14. Biederman J, Boellner SW, Childress A, Lopez FA, Krishna S, Zhang Y. Lisexamfetamine dimesyltate and mixed amphetamine salts extended-release in children with ADHD: a double-blind, placebo-controlled, crossover analog classroom study. *Biol Psychiatry*. 2007;62:970–976.

Further Reading

Arnsten AF. Catecholamine influences on dorsolateral prefrontal cortical networks. *Biol Psychiatry*. 2011;69:e89–e99.

Bidwell LC, Dew RE, Kollins SH. Alpha-2 adrenergic receptors and attention-deficit/hyperactivity disorder. *Curr Psychiatry Rep*. 2010;12:366–373.

Chapter 10

Clinical Medication Management

Key Points

- FDA-approved stimulants for ADHD are first-line pharmacotherapies followed by FDA-approved nonstimulants.
- Optimal medication titration promotes rapid symptom management and efficient use of clinical resources by assessing responses with the range of usual therapeutic doses over 2–3 weeks.
- Long-term adherence is enhanced by psychoeducation, patient and family participation in treatment decisions, and scheduling follow-up visits at regular intervals.
- Most side effects are easily managed by changes in medication, dose, or dosing schedule, or with combination pharmacotherapy.

In most cases, a diagnosis of ADHD leads to recommendations for pharmacotherapy (see Chapters 7 and 8). Although comprehensive treatment planning includes targeted academic, behavioral, and social interventions, only medication robustly addresses core ADHD symptoms. Pharmacotherapy is apt to be employed except in borderline or mild cases, with very young children, or if families are strongly opposed.

Initial Medication Selection

Medication selection follows an evidence-based approach. FDA-approved medications should be considered before those without ADHD indications. Stimulant medications have the largest treatment effects, largest number of placebo-controlled trials, longest history of use, and most accumulated safety data. Stimulants are easily titrated and with optimal doses effects are immediately evident. As such, practice algorithms for ADHD place stimulants as first-line therapies.[1-3]

Prior to use in a specific patient, all stimulants have the same potential benefits and risks (see Chapter 9). Initial stimulant choice should be tailored to individual patient needs and consider daily schedules and necessary effect duration, tolerability, compliance and ease of use, and patient/family preference. While research data suggest that methylphenidate (MPH) and

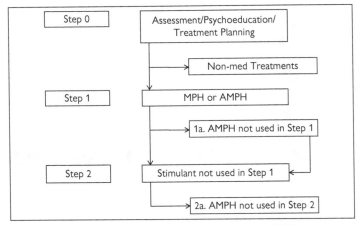

Figure 10.1 ADHD medication treatment algorithm, steps 0–2. AMPH, amphetamine; MPH, methylphenidate. (Adapted from Pliszka et al.[1])

amphetamine (AMPH) compounds have similar side effects, MPH is shown to be milder in meta-analysis.[4] As such, some prefer MPH initially in younger patients. Conversely, AMPH formulations might more reliably provide extended durations of effect required by older individuals. Whether or not a patient can swallow pills or capsules can bear on selection. Various medications might or might not be available on individual insurance formularies. Adequate consideration must be given to patient resources and ability to pay long-term prescription costs.

Initial steps for ADHD pharmacotherapy appear in Figure 10.1. Once an initial formulation of MPH or AMPH is chosen, the patient should be titrated on escalating doses within the standard therapeutic range over a 2- to 3-week period. If the medication is effective but has too long a duration of effect, for example, sleep is disturbed, a shorter acting form of the same stimulant might prove beneficial. If the initial choice does not provide sufficient improvement, or if there are problems with side effects or tolerability, a second trial with the alternative stimulant class (MPH or AMPH) should be initiated. There is little point in successive trials of different formulations of the same medication if one trial suggests it is ineffective or not tolerated. One exception is allowance for a second AMPH trial with the alternative AMPH, for example, mixed amphetamine salts (MAS) or lisdexamfetamine (LDX), not initially used, since some differences might emerge between mixed salts and prodrug AMPH.

The introduction of effective extended-release (ER) stimulants established once-daily dosing as the clinical standard.[5] Most clinicians begin titration with a once-daily ER stimulant, although some prefer an initial trial of an immediate-release (IR) form to confirm the patient can tolerate the drug. IR stimulants are commonly used to supplement once-daily ER forms to achieve a longer duration of clinical benefit (see Chapter 9). Some patients, particularly adults, prefer IR forms that allow them to restrict medication use to

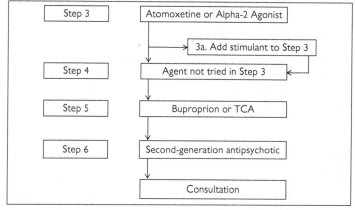

Figure 10.2 ADHD medication treatment algorithm, steps 3–6. TCA, tricyclic antidepressant. (Adapted from Pliszka et al.[1])

more limited periods of time. Others choose IR medication secondary to cost or insurance constraints.

FDA-approved nonstimulant medications are employed once a patient has failed stimulants (Fig. 10.2). More research data are available supporting use of atomoxetine than the ER alpha-2 agonists guanfacine and clonidine. This suggests that atomoxetine should be considered prior to the other nonstimulants. Atomoxetine may be considered first-line monotherapy for patients with comorbid tic or anxiety disorders. Nonstimulants may also be considered first-line treatments when there is high concern over potential stimulant misuse (see Chapters 11 and 12).

When monotherapy is partially effective or limited by side effects, combination stimulant and nonstimulant regimens can prove beneficial. Examples are combinations of MPH or AMPH with atomoxetine or alpha-2 agonists.[6,7] FDA approval has been granted for combination stimulant and ER alpha-2 agonist therapy, although combination therapy with stimulants and atomoxetine does not have FDA approval. Numerous agents without FDA approval are sometimes effective and typically used when approved medications fail, as adjunctive agents to augment treatment response, to address comorbidity, and when there is strong potential for stimulant misuse. Use of IR guanfacine and clonidine is substantially supported by research literature as well as FDA approval of the ER formulations. Other medications commonly prescribed off-label include modafinil, tricyclic antidepressants, buproprion, and certain antipsychotic agents. While some research evidence supports their use, efficacy data are limited and heightened attention to safety monitoring is advised.

Medication Titration

Following assessment and recommendations for pharmacotherapy, the initial medication trial should not be seen as provision of optimized treatment, but rather an opportunity to assess clinical response at various doses of the chosen drug in an individual patient. The goal of initial titration is to determine as quickly and efficiently as possible the optimal dose of an effective and well-tolerated medication. Generally, 5–7 days on a fixed stimulant dose is sufficient to assess treatment response and develop some tolerance to side effects. Shorter trials do not provide a sufficient sampling of response to attribute changes to medication effects. Longer trials, such as providing an initial prescription of a low-dose stimulant for 30 days or more, fail to assess potential benefits with higher doses and unnecessarily delay the time to achieving symptom improvement.

Medication titration can be constrained by local norms, clinician and patient time demands, and third-party payers. Insurance companies increasingly demand 30-day prescriptions for chronically administered medications and create obstacles for determination of optimal doses with an initial titration. Clinicians must devise titration methods that suit local circumstances, keeping in mind the need to assess a range of doses within a reasonable time frame.

One approach to stimulant titration is summarized in Table 10.1. Patients are provided with a prescription for a low dose of the chosen stimulant and instructed to take as directed. A written information sheet given to patients can direct them to take one tablet or capsule daily for the first 5 days, two for the second 5 days, and three for the third 5 days. In a slight variation for LDX titration, two prescriptions, one for 20 mg and one for 30 mg, are required. Medication should be taken all at once following breakfast. The information sheet should further direct patients to note their responses at various doses, summarize potential side effects, and request that they contact the physician's office if serious problems emerge. Absent significant difficulties, patients return for an office visit after 2–3 weeks to review responses and help the clinician determine which dose appears most effective and well tolerated. Clinicians may then provide a 30-day supply of the apparent best dose and schedule a 1-month follow-up visit to verify optimized response. If after the 1-month trial both patient and clinician are satisfied with treatment response, follow-up visits for ongoing stimulant management can be scheduled every 3 months. If a satisfactory medication and dose are not identified during initial titration, the process is repeated with a different agent.

Titration of nonstimulant medications follows a slightly different approach. Atomoxetine dosing is weight based with a target of 1.2–1.4 mg/kg per day and maximum of 100 mg per day. Problems with tolerability most frequently emerge when initial dose is too high or if doses are increased too quickly. Clinicians should initiate atomoxetine at 0.5 mg/kg or less per day for the initial week of therapy. If the dose is tolerated after 1 week, the dose may be doubled. This does not necessarily require an office assessment unless there are significant concerns about tolerability. Clinicians should assess response 1–2 weeks after the dose is doubled, and then increase to the full target dose if well tolerated. Atomoxetine can be taken once or twice daily in divided doses. Some benefit should be evident after a week at full dose, but improvements can continue to increase over several weeks. If there is insufficient improvement after a month at full dose, atomoxetine is unlikely to be beneficial and should be discontinued.

Table 10.1 Sample Stimulant Titration Regimens—Patient Is Given a Prescription Along With Written Instructions for How to Take

Medication/Dose	Number (#) Dispensed/ Script*	Patient Instructions
OROS-MPH 18 mg	#30	First 5 days: 1 tab
	1–2 qam as directed	Second 5 days: 2 tabs
		Third 5 days: 3 tabs
D-MPH-ER 5 mg	#30	First 5 days: 1 tab
Patient <25 kg	1–2 qam as directed	Second 5 days: 2 tabs
		Third 5 days: 3 tabs
D-MPH-ER 5 mg	#50	First 5 days: 2 tabs
Patient ≥25 kg	2–3 qam as directed	Second 5 days: 3 tabs
		Third 5 days: 4 tabs
MAS-ER 10 mg	#30	First 5 days: 1 tab
	1–2 qam as directed	Second 5 days: 2 tabs
		Third 5 days: 3 tabs
LDX 30 mg	#30	First 5 days:
Plus	1 qam as directed	1 X 30 mg
LDX 20 mg	#30	Second 5 days:
(two prescriptions given)	1–2 qam as directed	1 X 30 mg plus 1 X 20 mg
		Third 5 days:
		1 X 30 mg plus 2 X 20 mg

*Written scripts can be modified to meet local pharmacy/insurance requirements.

D-MPH, dexmethylphenidate; ER, extended release; LDX, isdexamfetamine; MAS, mixed amphetamine salts; MPH, methylphenidate; qam, each morning.

Limiting factors in titrating alpha-2 agonists are sedation and hypotension. Optimal titration requires weekly assessment of tolerability and symptom response until sufficient improvement is attained. Medication should be initiated at the lowest available dose and increased weekly by the same increment as tolerated. ER guanfacine is administered once daily, ER clonidine once or twice daily, IR guanfacine twice daily, and IR clonidine three times daily.

Combination Pharmacotherapy

It is preferable to keep medication regimens as simple as possible. However, combination pharmacotherapies are appropriately utilized to address residual symptoms, problems with tolerability and side effects, and comorbid disorders.[8] One commonly used combination is administering an IR stimulant in the afternoon to extend the duration of clinical benefit derived from an ER stimulant taken in the morning. In this instance, it is usually best to use the same medication in ER and IR forms, and to dose the IR at a level apt to maintain the same ascending plasma profile achieved with the morning ER

Table 10.2 Stimulant Release Profiles: Matching Extended-Release and Immediate-Release Doses

Drug	Dose	Equivalent	Afternoon IR Supplement
OROS-MPH	18 mg	MPH-IR 5 mg tid	MPH-IR 5 mg
(Concerta®)	36 mg	MPH-IR 10 mg tid	MPH-IR 10 mg
	54 mg	MPH-IR 15 mg tid	MPH-IR 15 mg
MPH-ER	10 mg	MPH-IR 5 mg bid	MPH-IR 5 mg
(Ritalin LA®)	20 mg	MPH-IR 10 mg bid	MPH-IR 10 mg
	40 mg	MPH-IR 20 mg bid	MPH-IR 20 mg
MPH-ER	10 mg	MPH-IR 3 mg am/7 mg noon	MPH-IR 10 mg
(Metadate CD®)	40 mg	MPH-IR 12 mg am/ 28mg noon	MPH-IR 30 mg
D-MPH-ER	5 mg	D-MPH-IR 2.5 mg bid	D-MPH-IR 2.5 mg
(Focalin XR®)	10 mg	D-MPH-IR 5 mg bid	D-MPH-IR 5 mg
	20 mg	D-MPH-IR 10 mg bid	D-MPH-IR 10 mg
MAS-ER	10 mg	MAS-IR 5 mg bid	MAS-IR 5 mg
(Adderall XR®)	20 mg	MAS-IR 10 mg bid	MAS-IR 10 mg
	30 mg	MAS-IR 15 mg bid	MAS-IR 15 mg
Lisdexamfetamine	30 mg	MAS-XR 10 mg	MAS-IR 5 mg
(Vyvanse ®)	50 mg	MAS-XR 20 mg	MAS-IR 10 mg
	70 mg	MAS-XR 30 mg	MAS-IR15 mg

bid, twice daily morning and noon; D-MPH, dexmethylphenidate; ER, extended release; IR, immediate release; MAS, mixed amphetamine salts; MPH, methylphenidate; tid, three times daily.

dose (Table 10.2) (see Chapter 9). Stimulant and nonstimulant combinations are often useful when stimulant doses require reduction due to weight loss or when addressing tic exacerbations, rebound hyperactivity, late afternoon irritability, and sleep difficulties. With the exception of stimulants and ER alpha-2 agonists in treating treatment refractory ADHD symptoms, these combinations are considered off-label uses.

Long-Term Maintenance

Once an apparently optimal medication and dose have been identified, it is advisable to provide a 1-month prescription and then reassess to confirm that symptoms are adequately controlled. After the clinician and patient agree that clinical needs are well addressed, subsequent follow-up visits can be scheduled every 3 months. Assessment of height, weight, pulse, and blood pressure can be limited to every 6 months.[9] Some clinicians are content to provide long-term refills without requiring patient appointments and only reassess patients as needed. This is not an acceptable standard of care.

As with all chronic conditions, patient adherence with prescribed treatment is improved by regular clinical contact and active inclusion of patients and families in their medical decision making.[10] Clinical improvement is best maintained with regular monitoring and dose adjustments, likely to be required as the patient grows. Clinicians are not able to assist with ongoing management if not regularly apprised of patient needs. Regular assessment facilitates initiation of family, academic, and social interventions as needed. Treatment compliance is further improved with more extensive evaluation and provision of appropriate education about the disorder.[10]

Finally, the US Drug Enforcement Agency (DEA) only allows up to a 90-day prescription of Schedule II drugs and requires clinical reassessment before additional refills can be provided. Depending on the patient's insurance plan, clinicians can write for a single 90-day supply or provide three separate prescriptions for 30-day supplies, with notations that prescriptions not be filled until 1 and 2 months later for the second and third prescriptions, respectively. Nonstimulant medications are not limited to 90-day supplies and can be renewed without clinical reassessment. However, patients still benefit from consistent and regularly scheduled follow-up visits for the other reasons described. Careful documentation of all prescribed medications is essential.

Managing Common Side Effects

Most side effects to ADHD medication are mild to moderate in severity. General management strategies include changes in dose or dose forms, switching to alternative medications, or combination drug treatments. Medications that cause unacceptable side effects or are not tolerated must be discontinued.

Appetite Loss and Growth Delay

It is advisable to anticipate appetite loss and recommend calorie supplementation when stimulant therapy is initiated, not after weight loss occurs. Medication is best taken after eating breakfast and other meals, and late evening meals and high-caloric snacks should be encouraged. Appetite, height, weight, and body mass index should be assessed at least every 6 months.[9] It is important to differentiate baseline "picky" eating from stimulant-related appetite suppression and parental concerns about decreased appetite from documented weight losses. Loss of 5% or more body weight from baseline or failure to gain height or weight over a year should be addressed with stimulant dose reductions, switch to shorter acting stimulant or alternative drug class, or medication holidays on weekends and vacations.[11] Children who exhibit deceleration of growth rate usually make up their growth losses once medication is discontinued (see Chapter 12). Medication holidays over two, but not one, summer vacations promote successful recovery from lost growth. Children at or below the 3rd percentile for height at a given age should be referred for evaluation by a pediatric endocrinologist.

Headache, Stomachache, Nausea

It can be difficult to determine whether headache, stomachache, nausea, and other somatic complaints are caused by medication or underlying ADHD. In many studies, these effects occur equally in children taking active stimulants or placebo.[12] Management approaches include on-off-on medications trials, dose reductions, taking medication with food, and switching to alternative medication. These side effects are particularly common with atomoxetine and alpha-2 agonists, and they can respond to dose reductions. Palliative treatment, such as acetaminophen or ibuprofen for headache, can be considered and used if effective in relieving symptoms. A change in medication class or abandonment of pharmacotherapy might be necessary if these symptoms persist at intolerable levels.

Mood Lability and Irritability

It is important to differentiate mood changes that span the entire day from briefer "rebound" episodes that occur in the late afternoon when stimulant effects are wearing off. With pervasive mood changes, the possibility of comorbid mood or anxiety disorders should be reconsidered. Atomoxetine can be preferentially beneficial in individuals exhibiting stimulant-related mood changes. Serotonin reuptake inhibitors (SRIs) might be indicated as adjunctive stimulant treatment with evidence of depression, anxiety, or chronic irritability.[1]

Psychosis

True psychotic symptoms are rare with ADHD medications. The most typical psychotic symptom attributable to stimulants is formication, the sense that insects are crawling under the skin. The first step when psychotic symptoms emerge is to confirm that the patient is not exceeding therapeutic drug doses. Lowering the medication dose or stopping medication altogether allows determination of whether symptoms cease or persist. If psychotic symptoms resolve, a medication rechallenge at the previous dose can establish whether the psychosis is related to drug effects. Persistent psychotic symptoms necessitate additional diagnostic clarification.

Rebound Hyperactivity

Many individuals on stimulant therapy have persistent adverse reactions in mid- to late afternoon when medication effects are waning. These can include increased mood lability, irritability, hyperactivity and restlessness, and fatigue. Several strategies to assess this difficulty can be tried on a case-by-case basis. These include switching to a longer acting or alternative stimulant, addition of a nonstimulant, or switching to nonstimulant monotherapy. Ensuring that the child has a balanced snack after school can also prove helpful, particularly when lunch is skipped due to appetite loss or other reasons.

Sleep Difficulties

Many individuals with ADHD have sleep difficulties, on or off medication.[9] A typical picture is that ADHD patients have severe problems settling to bed in the evening, but once asleep they are very difficult to arouse. It is essential to document baseline sleep patterns prior to initiation of medication. Sleep laboratory assessment might be indicated if there are suspicions of sleep apnea, episodic nocturnal phenomena, excessive limb movements, or unexplained daytime drowsiness. Proper sleep hygiene, including the implementation of a standard bedtime routine and minimal use of electronics after dinner, must be emphasized prior to any changes in pharmacotherapy. Once sleep difficulties are clearly attributed to ADHD medication, options might include addition of a low-dose short-acting stimulant in the evening to counteract rebound hyperactivity, switching to a shorter acting stimulant formulation for morning administration, or adjunctive treatment with an IR alpha-2 agonists given after dinner or twice daily. Melatonin is useful for some patients, but care must be taken to ensure that only pharmaceutical grade drug is administered.

Suicidality

Suicidal thoughts and behaviors are extremely rare during ADHD pharmacotherapy. Their emergence suggests the existence of comorbid psychiatric disorders or severe psychosocial stress.[9] As with psychosis, it might be useful to assess symptoms after lowering doses or discontinuing medication, but absent any clear relationship with suicidal symptoms, there is no contraindication to continuing ADHD treatment.

Discontinuing Medication

While it is undeniable that ADHD medications provide short-term benefits, evidence supporting positive effects on long-term functioning beyond symptom control remains limited.[13] Many patients and families discontinue medication on their own, providing immediate evidence about whether ongoing treatment is warranted. Alternatively, scheduled breaks from medication are also helpful in determining whether pharmacotherapy remains justified. Decisions over starting, continuing, or discontinuing medication must be individualized. Clinicians remain obligated on at least an annual basis to reassess relative benefits and risks of sustained pharmacotherapy.

References

1. Pliszka SR, Crismon ML, Hughes CW, et al. The Texas Children's Medication Algorithm Project: revision of the algorithm for pharmacotherapy of attention-deficit//hyperactivity disorder. *J Am Acad Child Adolesc Psychiatry.* 2006;45:642–667.

2. Subcommittee on Attention-Deficit/Hyperactivity Disorder, Steering Committee on Quality Improvement and Management. ADHD: clinical practice guidelines for the diagnosis, evaluation, and treatment of attention-deficit/hyperactivity disorder in children and adolescents. *Pediatrics.* 2011;128;1007–1022.

3. Kooij SJ, Bejerot S, Blackwell A, et al. European consensus statement on diagnosing and treatment of adult ADHD: The European Network Adult ADHD. *BMC Psychiatry.* 2010;67.

4. Faraone SV, Buitelaar J. Comparing the efficacy of stimulants for ADHD in children and adolescents using met-analysis. *Eur Child Adolesc Psychiatry.* 2010;19:353–364.

5. Biederman J, Spencer T. Psychopharmacological interventions. *Child Adolesc Psychiatry Clin N Am.* 2008;17:439–458.

6. Wilens TE, Bukstein O, Brams M, et al. A controlled trial of extended-release guanfacine and psychostimulants for attention-deficit/hyperactivity disorder. *J Am Acad Child Adolesc Psychiatry*. 2012;51:74–85.

7. Treuer T, Gau SS, Médez L, et al. A systematic review of combination therapy with stimulants and atomoxetine for attention-deficit/hyperactivity disorder, including patient characteristics, treatment strategies, effectiveness, and tolerability. *J Child Adolesc Psychopharmacol*. 2013;23:179–193.

8. Wilens TE. Combined pharmacotherapy in pediatric psychopharmacology: friend or foe? *J Child Adolesc Psychopharmacol*. 2009;19:484–484.

9. Cortese S, Holtmann M, Banaschewski T, et al. Practitioner review: current best practice in the management of adverse events during treatment with ADHD medications in children and adolescents. *J Child Psychol Psychiatry*. 2013:54:227–246.

10. Charach A, Fernandez R. Enhancing ADHD medication adherence: challenges and opportunities. *Curr Psychiatry Rep*. 2013;15:371.

11. Martins S, Tramontina S, Polanczyk G, et al. Weekend holidays during methylphenidate use in ADHD children: a randomized clinical trial. *J Child Adolesc Psychopharmacol*. 2004;14:195–205.

12. Barkley RA, McMurray MB, Edelbrock CS, Robbins K. Side effects of methylphenidate in children with attention deficit hyperactivity disorder: a systemic, placebo-controlled evaluation. *Pediatrics*. 1990;86:184–192.

13. Van de Loo-Neus GH, Rommelse N, Buitelaar JK. To stop or not to stop: how long should medication treatment of attention-deficit hyperactivity disorder be extended? *Eur Neuropsychopharmacol*. 2011;21:584–599.

Further Reading

McBurnett K, Swetye M, Muhr H, Hendren RL. Pharmacotherapy of inattention and ADHD in adolescents. *Adolesc Med State Art Rev*. 2013;24:391–405.

Riddle MA, dosReis S, Reeves GM, Wissow LS, Preitt DB, Foy JM. Pediatric psychopharmacology in primary care: a conceptual framework. *Adolesc Med State Art Rev*. 2013;24:371–390.

Wilens TE, Morrison NR, Prince J. An update on the pharmacotherapy of attention-deficit/hyperactivity in adults. *Expert Rev Neurother*. 2011;11:1443–1465.

Chapter 11

Comorbidity

Key Points

- Comorbidity is common with ADHD.
- ADHD treatment frequently requires concurrent management of other disorders.

Potential comorbidity should be considered during initial ADHD evaluations and whenever treatment response is unsatisfactory (see Chapter 6). Given limited resources, clinicians must carefully integrate the range of treatments necessary to relieve both ADHD and co-occurring disorders. This includes pharmacotherapy as well as numerous behavioral and psychosocial interventions with evidence supporting their utility for specific conditions (Box 11.1).

Disruptive Behavior Disorders

Oppositional defiant disorder (ODD) and conduct disorder (CD) are the most common co-occurring conditions in pediatric ADHD, approaching 50% lifetime prevalence.[1] ODD is typified by frequent and persistent patterns of angry or irritable mood, argumentative and defiant behavior, and vindictiveness. CD is characterized by persistent behaviors that violate either basic rights of others or major age-appropriate social norms.

Virtually all children with ODD or CD have ADHD. Between 30% and 50% of ODD is evident by age 5.[2] Recent research suggests that ODD comprises two distinct dimensions, with irritable mood symptoms predicting subsequent depression and anxiety, and argumentative/defiant behaviors predicting subsequent conduct disorder.[3] As with ADHD, the severity and frequency of ODD symptoms must exceed what is developmentally expected. For example, occasional temper outbursts and defiance are common in preschoolers and would not indicate the diagnosis. Symptoms cannot be limited to struggles over schoolwork related to ADHD or other learning impairments. In older youth, particularly in families with strict cultural expectations, parental concerns about oppositional behaviors and defiance must be balanced against general societal norms as well as the individual's maturity level and emerging independence. In most cases, ODD remits by mid to late adolescence.

Distinctions between childhood- and adolescent-onset CD are long noted. Childhood-onset CD requires emergence of at least one symptom by age 10.

Box 11.1 Evidenced-Based Behavioral and Psychosocial Treatments

General
Psychoeducation

Disruptive Behavior Disorders
Behavioral contracting
Contingency management
Multisystemic therapy (MST)
Parent management training

Learning Disorders
Academic accommodations

Substance Use Disorders
Cognitive-behavioral therapy (CBT)
Multidimensional family therapy (MDFT)

Anxiety Disorders
CBT
Exposure therapy
Exposure/response prevention

Depression
CBT
Interpersonal psychotherapy (IPT)

Bipolar Disorders
Family-focused treatment (FFT)

Tic Disorders
Habit reversal therapy (HRT)

Childhood-onset CD is almost always preceded by ADHD and ODD, although the majority of children do not subsequently develop CD. Childhood onset predicts significantly more lifetime pathology, including higher rates of school and occupational failure, substance use difficulties, aggression, and antisocial behaviors. The worst outcomes associated with ADHD are largely mediated by CD. Children with ADHD and childhood-onset CD typically have lower socioeconomic status and higher rates of antisocial and aggressive behaviors among first-degree family members.[1] Conversely, only a third of individuals with adolescent-onset CD exhibit co-occurring ADHD. Adolescent onset is more usually time limited, associated with acute psychosocial stress, and less likely to include significant aggression or inadequate development of peer relationships.

Stimulants are effective in treating ODD and CD, apart from independent improvements in ADHD. ODD symptoms also respond to atomoxetine and alpha-2 agonists. Stimulants improve compliance with parental demands and reduce overt and covert aggression, lying, stealing, and vandalism. Limited evidence suggests that lithium and divalproex sodium are better than placebo in controlling aggressive outbursts, but they are ineffective for ADHD.[1] Several studies suggest some role for second-generation antipsychotic medications, particularly risperidone, in controlling irritability and aggression.[2] However, these carry significant risks for weight gain, metabolic syndrome, and other adverse outcomes. None of these are currently FDA-approved uses.

Psychosocial interventions are often important in managing ODD and CD, whether or not pharmacotherapy is employed. The same psychosocial and behavioral treatments recommended for ADHD, particularly parent management training, are useful with ODD (see Chapter 7). For older children, parent management approaches can give way to negotiation of behavioral contracts that establish clear behavioral expectations and consequences. Some older children also benefit from cognitive interventions that teach improved problem solving, communication, social skills, and impulse control. New evidence suggests that multifamily psychoeducational psychotherapy (MF-PEP), developed for treatment of mood disorders, might have similarly positive effects for ODD, but not CD.[4]

CD interventions are difficult and expensive. Treatment, including pharmacotherapy if indicated, should be initiated for any identifiable comorbid disorder, such as ADHD, depression, anxiety, or substance use. CD is often associated with high levels of family chaos. This suggests it is best to emphasize behaviorally focused, time-limited interventions that teach clear guidelines for parental responses toward their children's behaviors. Multisystemic therapy (MST) is a type of parent management training that provides a comprehensive approach to family, marital, academic, and peer-related issues. MST has proven useful in controlled trials, but it is expensive, time intensive, and not widely available. Less specialized patient-based cognitive approaches and parent management strategies are also used, but they are not supported by a substantial evidence base.

Group therapies, which increase exposure to other youth with severe behavioral difficulties, as well as individual psychodynamic or psychoanalytic therapies, or open-ended family treatments, are generally regarded as ineffective interventions for disruptive behavior disorders.

Learning Disorders

Between 10% and 50% of individuals with ADHD have specific learning disorders.[2] Learning disorders are defined by persistent difficulties acquiring critical academic skills combined with academic achievement levels that are substantially below expectations for the student's age or developmental level. Specific learning disorders in reading, spelling, and mathematics appear to have some genetic basis, but they are also influenced by family and environmental factors. Assessment requires administration of standardized tests that allow comparisons of intellectual ability with academic performance.

ADHD medications can enhance success on academic tests, although there are no FDA-approved medication treatments for learning disability. Remedial tutoring can improve academic skills, particularly when individualized approaches to learning are incorporated. Academic accommodations, including preferential classroom seating, modified work assignments, note-taking services, and additional time on standardized tests can be implemented under individualized education plans (IEPs) (see Chapters 7 and 8).

Substance Use Disorders

Compared with unaffected youth, individuals with ADHD are more likely to experiment with psychoactive substances at younger ages and develop problems related to substance use.[5] Lifetime prevalence estimates of substance use disorders in ADHD range from 20% to 25% for adolescents and 45% to 55% for adults. Suggestions that substance use represents attempts at self-medicating ADHD have not been borne out by research. The most commonly used psychoactive substances are nicotine, alcohol, and cannabis, which reflect societal patterns. Numerous studies confirm that ADHD treatment does not increase subsequent risk for substance use difficulties, nor does ADHD pharmacotherapy during childhood and adolescence reduce future substance use risk.[5] More severe substance use disorders are generally associated with a history of conduct disorder.

It is critically important to document the nature and extent of psychoactive substance in patients with ADHD. Core features of substance use disorders include impaired control of use, social impairment, risky behaviors, or features of tolerance or withdrawal. Substance use is not equal to substance use disorder. For example, it could be argued that occasional recreational use of alcohol or marijuana is normative in some age groups and not associated with any of these core features described. Individuals reporting intermittent recreational alcohol or marijuana use are likely to be very different than those with daily cocaine or opiate use. Recognition of these differences is critical for effective treatment planning.

Clinicians should differentiate substance use and use disorders from misuse and diversion. Misuse is use of a substance for a purpose other than which it was intended. One-time recreational use of a prescription drug is not misuse unless criteria for a substance use disorder are also met. Diversion is the transfer of prescription medication from one person to another, regardless of subsequent use. Patients with comorbid conduct or substance use disorders have increased risks for misuse and diversion of prescription ADHD medications.

There is no clear consensus on clinical management of patients with ADHD and comorbid substance use disorders (see Chapter 12). In addition to quantifying substance use, it is essential for clinicians to very carefully document specific target symptoms, treatment responses, and doses and quantities of medication provided with each prescription. Some physicians refuse to prescribe medication for adult ADHD due to concerns about potential abuse and misuse. This is an extreme position. In contrast, although stimulants are contraindicated for concomitant use with other psychoactive drugs, many physicians are comfortable prescribing them despite occasional recreational use of alcohol or cannabis. Nonstimulant ADHD medications are acceptable alternatives if the provider determines there is too much risk with a stimulant prescription. As substance use disorders increase in severity, clinical emphasis generally shifts from ADHD to substance use. There is no evidence that ADHD medications worsen co-occurring substance use or increase success of substance use treatment.

Anxiety Disorders

Approximately one third of children and up to half of adults with ADHD have clinically significant anxiety.[1] Many meet full diagnostic criteria for social phobia, generalized anxiety disorder, and, in youth, separation anxiety disorder. Others suffer substantial anxiety-related impairments but do not strictly meet specific categorical criteria. Anxious children with ADHD have more school- and peer-related difficulties than those with ADHD alone. Families of these children exhibit higher rates of marital difficulties, separations, and divorce.

Several early stimulant studies described decreased symptom responses and increased adverse event rates in anxious children with ADHD, suggesting that anxiety is a contraindication for stimulant therapy. Other reports fail to support this view. Numerous and more recent controlled studies demonstrate that children with and without anxiety have similar rates of stimulant-related ADHD response. In the Multimodal Treatment Study of ADHD (MTA), 34% of participants had clinically significant anxiety. Anxiety was not associated with worse outcomes, and many participants had meaningful reductions in anxiety with stimulant monotherapy. Anxious children were more likely to benefit from combination medication and psychosocial interventions than those with ADHD alone.[6] It has been proposed that anxious children and their families might be more treatment adherent when provided additional support through parent management and other psychosocial interventions, but this has not been tested scientifically. In a pilot study based on MTA findings, participants with ADHD and comorbid anxiety disorders were initially titrated on a stimulant to reduce ADHD symptoms and then randomized to fluvoxamine or placebo.[7] About 10% had clinically significant reductions in anxiety with stimulant alone. Those subsequently randomized to fluvoxamine showed a trend for improved anxiety, although this did not meet statistical significance in the small sample. In a randomized controlled study atomoxetine was effective for both ADHD and anxiety; however, atomoxetine is not FDA approved as an anxiety medication.

Based on these and other studies, one approach to medication management is to initiate stimulant treatment (Fig. 11.1). Given that stimulants can be titrated quickly, this often allows for rapid improvement in ADHD, and some individuals might also have significant reductions in anxiety. In those with ongoing anxiety-related impairment, combination therapy with a selective serotonin reuptake inhibitor can be initiated. An alternative approach is to initiate treatment with a nonstimulant, either atomoxetine or an alpha-2 agonist, that might be effective for both ADHD and anxiety symptoms (Fig. 11.2). Again, however, neither of these medications has an FDA indication for anxiety treatment.

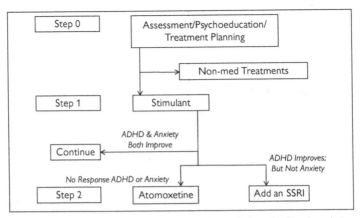

Figure 11.1 Treatment algorithm for ADHD and comorbid anxiety disorders; choice to begin with stimulant. SSRI, selective serotonin reuptake inhibitor. (Adapted from Pliszka et al.[13])

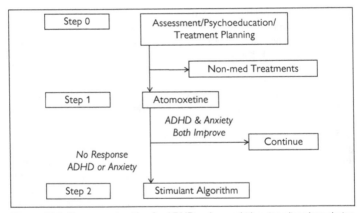

Figure 11.2 Treatment algorithm for ADHD and comorbid anxiety disorders; choice to begin with nonstimulant. (Adapted from Pliszka et al.[13])

Parents of anxious children are often anxious themselves and might be more reluctant than others to accept recommendations for pharmacotherapy. Patients with anxiety are often more prone to experience medication-related side effects. In general, a conservative approach that uses lower initial medication doses and more gradual dose titrations, particularly with an SSRI, promotes greater acceptance of treatment with gradual exposure. Other psychosocial approaches to anxiety disorders, particularly psychoeducational and cognitive-behavioral therapies, are often useful with this group.

Depression

Over their lifetimes, 20% of individuals with ADHD have at least one episode of major depression.[2] Depression is two to three times greater in

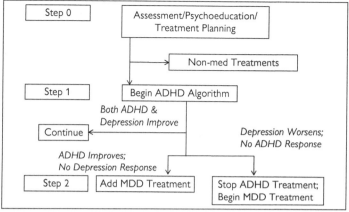

Figure 11.3 Treatment algorithm for ADHD and comorbid depression; ADHD more impairing. MDD, major depressive disorder. (Adapted from Pliszka et al.[13])

ADHD-affected youth. Precise rates of juvenile depression can be difficult to determine because parents and children often differ in reported symptoms. Many depressive symptoms are not disorder specific. Concentration deficits are seen in mood and anxiety disorders as well as ADHD. Irritability is a core feature of juvenile depression, oppositional defiant disorder, and disruptive mood dysregulation disorder. Some youth appear depressed and anhedonic when frustrated about school or punished for some aspect of their behavior, but they are readily engaged and motivated to participate in nonacademic or social activities. Some view this picture as evidence of demoralization and not depression. In other cases, particularly with persistent low mood, sleep or appetite disturbances, decreased energy distinct from usual functioning, or excessive guilt and low self-esteem, depression is more likely.

A general approach to treatment of ADHD and comorbid depression is to determine initially which condition is more impairing. With demoralization or milder depression, initial stimulant treatment can rapidly improve ADHD symptoms and related feelings of failure and other mood symptoms (Fig. 11.3). Subsequent antidepressant therapy is appropriate in those with lingering mood-related difficulties. In cases dominated by low mood, particularly with any degree of suicidality, it is typically better to initiate appropriate treatment for depression, possibly including both therapy and antidepressant medication (Fig. 11.4). Adjunctive stimulant medication can be initiated if ADHD persists subsequent to resolution of mood symptoms. An alternative to this sequential approach is to utilize a medication that might improve both ADHD and depression. Buproprion has been proved effective in both juvenile and adult ADHD and is useful in adult depression, although it is not FDA approved for ADHD. A study of atomoxetine in pediatric patients showed ADHD improvement but no antidepressant response. Atomoxetine and subsequent combination therapy with fluoxetine appears effective for ADHD and depression.[8]

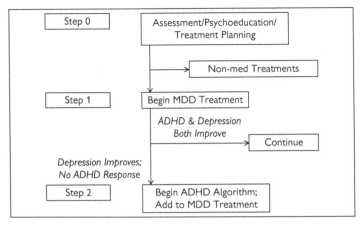

Figure 11.4 Treatment algorithm for ADHD and comorbid depression; depression more impairing. MDD, major depressive disorder. (Adapted from Pliszka et al.[13])

The potential role of psychotherapy for depression treatment should not be ignored. There is a strong evidence base for cognitive-behavioral therapy and interpersonal psychotherapy, among others, for both juvenile and adult depression. Medication is appropriately used with persistent or more severe depressive episodes, when daily mood symptoms occurring more often than not, or with associated problems with sleep, appetite, or suicidality. Several selective serotonin reuptake inhibitors (SSRIs) are indicated for pediatric depression, although treatment effect sizes are not as large as with adults. Combination strategies that integrate appropriate therapy and medication are usually most effective in children and adolescents. SSRIs are not useful for ADHD symptoms. There is a small potential for interactions between some SSRIs and stimulants due to genetic variability in metabolic pathways, but these are rarely significant clinically.

Bipolar Disorders

There is long-standing controversy on the purported co-occurrence of ADHD and bipolar disorder. Some studies concluded that 20% of children with ADHD also met criteria for mania.[9] Unlike adults who typically exhibit discrete episodes of euphoria and grandiosity, these children and adolescents were more likely to exhibit chronic difficulties with irritability and hyper-arousal. Subsequent research determined, among other differences, that children with chronic irritability were more likely as young adults to be diagnosed with ADHD and depression, while those with episodic irritability had higher lifetime risks for psychosis, subsequent manic episodes, and a parent with classic bipolar disorder.[10] *DSM-5* criteria for bipolar disorder clarify that manic symptoms must occur within distinct episodes that depart from usual behavior. This clarification eliminated the bipolar diagnosis in individuals with a defining feature of chronic irritability.

Given past inconsistencies in the application of *DSM* bipolar criteria in youth with ADHD, reliable estimates of comorbidity are unknown. Based on *DSM-5*, clinicians must carefully distinguish ADHD symptoms, which are expected to have childhood onset, persistent duration, and may or may not be associated with chronic irritability, from acute-onset manic symptoms that occur during discrete episodes with associated changes in mood, sleep, overactivity, distractibility, or risk taking that clearly differs from usual functioning. While comorbidity rates of bipolar disorder and ADHD may not be as high as previously thought, clinicians should remain alert to their possible co-occurrence.

When present, manic symptoms must be controlled using a standard mood stabilizer or second-generation antipsychotic. Lithium, aripiprazole, and risperidone are approved treatments for mania in children aged 10 years and older. Off-label therapies, including use of these medications in younger patients as well as divalproex sodium, are also employed, although evidence supporting their use is scant. Once euthymia is attained, a stimulant can be added to mood-stabilizing therapy to address residual ADHD. Several studies have shown that adding stimulants to either lithium or divalproex is safe and leads to improvement in ADHD compared with placebo.[1] Careful monitoring for potential exacerbations of mania or psychosis is essential. Alternatively, an initial stimulant trial under close supervision is acceptable with an uncertain history of mania, as severe ADHD symptoms are sometimes confused for bipolar disorder. Long-term stimulant use does not appear to increase risk for mania provided that treatment antimanic therapy is sustained.

Disruptive Mood Dysregulation Disorder

Early definitions of ADHD included affective instability and irritability as core features, although these were removed from *DSM-III* and subsequent criteria. Some aspects of chronic irritability and related difficulties were incorporated into criteria for oppositional defiant disorder. Research on chronic irritability initiated in response to questions about juvenile bipolar disorder proposed a category called severe mood dysregulation (SMD), defined by frequent and severe temper outbursts, persistent irritable or angry mood, and symptoms of hyperarousal such as insomnia, distractibility, or intrusiveness. Individuals with SMD have distinct biological and cognitive profiles, and increased risk for ADHD, mood, and anxiety disorders.[11] This research led to inclusion in *DSM-5* of disruptive mood dysregulation disorder (DMDD), a new diagnostic category defined similarly to SMD without the requirement for hyperarousal. Research on rates of co-occurring DMDD and ADHD, as well as optimal approaches to treatment, remains limited. The ultimate utility of DMDD as a diagnostic category has not been determined.

Despite uncertainties in nomenclature, a clear subset of individuals with ADHD manifests chronic irritability and associated temper outbursts or aggressive episodes. Treatment with second-generation antipsychotic agents, such as risperidone or ziprasidone, decreases irritability and aggression but is associated with serious side effects. None of these medication treatments has an FDA indication for this use. Some research on SMD suggests that stimulant treatment with adjunctive SSRI therapy might be a better tolerated and more optimal approach to DMDD, but this requires additional study. Family-based behavioral therapies are potentially important, particularly those that incorporate cognitive-behavioral approaches to affective regulation. Substantial research is required before definitive recommendations regarding comorbid DMDD can be made.

Tic Disorders

Motor tics, that is, rapid, recurrent, involuntary movements, are common and often unnoticed. Tic disorders, including both motor and vocal tics, require symptom persistence for at least 1 year and are associated with varying levels of distress and impairment. Tics typically have onset before puberty and most commonly decrease in frequency and severity during adolescence. Approximately 10% of children with ADHD have tic disorders—much higher than seen in the general population. Some have proposed genetic relationships between the two disorders.

Tics naturally wax and wane and shift affected muscle groups and vocalizations over time. Episodic exacerbations often alternate with periods of relief. Tic disorders were once considered absolute contraindication for stimulant treatment. Current meta-analyses reveal that long-term stimulant treatment has little overall impact on tic expression.[12]

Current recommendations suggest that stimulants remain first-line ADHD therapies, even in the presence of tics. If a clear exacerbation of tics occurs following treatment initiation, an alternative class of stimulants can be tried. If the second stimulant is also associated with increased tics, a switch to a nonstimulant ADHD medication is warranted. Nonstimulants are also acceptable as initial therapies, although the ADHD response is generally less robust than seen with stimulants. Atomoxetine has no impact on tics but is effective for ADHD. Alpha-2 agonists are shown to reduce tics and improve ADHD, although these are off-label treatments. Combination therapies, in particular, adding an alpha-2 agonist to a stimulant, can be especially effective and can provide additional ADHD benefit as well as tic control. If tics remain severe and refractory, first-generation antipsychotics such as haloperidol or pimozide, which have FDA approval as tic therapies, or second-generation agents such as risperidone or ziprasidone, which do not have an FDA indication, may be justified. Adjunctive treatment with habit reversal therapy, a cognitive-behavioral treatment shown to be effective in reducing tics, can be a useful component of overall management.

References

1. Pliszka S. Psychiatric comorbidities in children with attention deficit hyperactivity disorder. *Pediatr Drugs*. 2003;5:742–750.

2. Spencer TJ. Issues in the management of patients with complex attention-deficit/hyperactivity symptoms. *CNS Drugs*. 2009;23:9–20.

3. Burke JD, Hipwell AE, Loeber R. Dimensions of oppositional defiant disorder as predictors of depression and conduct disorder in preadolescent girls. *J Am Acad Child Adolesc Psychiatry*. 2010;119:49:484–492.

4. Boylan K, Macpherson HA, Fristad MA. Examination of disruptive behavior outcomes and moderation in a randomized psychotherapy trial for mood disorders. *J Am Acad Child Adolesc Psychiatry*. 2013;52:699–708.

5. Wilens TE, Martelon M, Joshi G, et al. Does ADHD predict substance-use disorders? A 10-year follow-up study of young adults with ADHD. *J Am Acad Child Adolesc Psychiatry*. 2011;50:543–553.

6. March JS, Swanson JM, Arnold LE, et al. Anxiety as a predictor and outcome variable in the multimodal treatment study of children with ADHD (MTA). *J Abnorm Child Psychol*. 2000;28:527–541.

7. Abikoff H, McGough J, Vitiello B, et al. Sequential pharmacotherapy for children with comorbid attention-deficit/hyperactivity and anxiety disorders. *J Am Acad Child Adolesc Psychiatry*. 2005;44:418–427.

8. Kratochvil CJ, Newcorn JH, Arnold LE, et al. Atomoxetine alone or combined with fluoxetine for treating ADHD with comorbid depressive or anxiety symptoms. *J Am Acad Child Adolesc Psychiatry*. 2005;44:915–924.

9. Wozniak J, Biederman J, Kiely K, et al. Mania-like symptoms suggestive of childhood-onset bipolar disorder in clinically referred children. *J Am Acad Child Adolesc Psychiatry*. 1995;34:867–876.

10. Brotman MA, Schmajuk M, Rich BA, et al. Prevalence, clinical correlates, and longitudinal course of severe mood dysregulation in children. *Biol Psychiatry*. 2006;60:991–997.

11. Leibenluft E. Severe mood dysregulation, irritability, and the diagnostic boundaries of bipolar disorder in youths. *Am J Psychiatry*. 2011;168:129–142.

12. Bloch MH, Panza KE, Landeros-Weisenberger A, Lechman JF. Meta-analysis: treatment of attention-deficit/hyperactivity disorder in children with comorbid tic disorders. *J Am Acad Child Adolesc Psychiatry*. 2009;48:884–893.

13. Pliszka SR, Crismon ML, Hughes CW, et al. The Texas Children's Medication Algorithm Project: revision of the algorithm for pharmacotherapy of attention-deficit/hyperactivity disorder. *J Am Acad Chlld Adolesc Psychiatry*. 2006;45:642–657.

Further Reading

Bond DJ, Hadjipavlou G, Lam RW, et al. The Canadian Network for Mood and Anxiety Treatments (CANMAT) task force recommendations for the management of patients with mood disorders and comorbid attention-deficit/hyperactivity disorder. *Ann Clin Psychiatry*. 2012;24:23–37.

Upadhyaya HP. Managing attention-deficit/hyperactivity disorder in the presence of substance use disorder. *J Clin Psychiatry*. 2007; 68:23–30.

Chapter 12

Medication Controversies

Key Points

- Medications for ADHD have been used for over 70 years and are widely regarded as safe and effective.
- ADHD medications have some side effect risks that must be balanced against potential treatment benefits.
- Some serious concerns about the safety of ADHD medications have no factual basis.

ADHD medications have been widely used for over 70 years (see Chapter 2). Despite hundreds of clinical trials demonstrating efficacy and safety, as well as epidemiological evidence resulting from millions of prescriptions written annually, recurrent concerns about these medications persist among medical professionals and the lay public. This chapter summarizes information on common controversies surrounding ADHD pharmacotherapy.

Do ADHD Medications Stunt Growth?

Ongoing debate continues as to whether ADHD medications cause delayed growth and decreased height. These concerns arise from the well-recognized appetite suppressive and weight loss effects of stimulants, as well as known inhibitory effects of increased synaptic dopamine on growth hormone. Although only some patients lose significant weight during stimulant treatment, virtually all clinical trials have shown that children fail to make expected gains in weight and height, particularly during the earliest period of treatment.[1] Growth delays appear greatest in younger versus older youth and in children who are taller and heavier than age-matched peers. Growth rates in early adolescence appear to be unaffected.

Numerous investigations have compared growth trajectories in medicated and never-medicated children, as well as typically developing youth without ADHD.[1] Stimulants are clearly associated with decreased growth velocity, with gains in height and weight less than expected for a given age. At the point of greatest deficit, these children are on average 2 cm shorter than nonmedicated peers. Stimulant-treated patients continue to grow, but more slowly than anticipated. Growth decelerations are most significant during the first 18 months but attenuate with ongoing treatment. The MTA

Study found greatest deficits in growth velocity during year 1, decreased deficits in year 2, and normalization by year 3.[2] Similarly, other investigations suggest that height deficits are greatest during the first 6 months of treatment but decrease over time.[1] Growth deficits are smaller in individuals with previous stimulant trials, providing further evidence that these effects diminish with ongoing therapy. Importantly, children appear to reach expected sizes within 2 years of treatment cessation, and several studies indicate that ultimate adult height is not affected. Similar patterns are seen in clinical trials of atomoxetine.[3]

Other research is less consistent.[1] Some reports suggest greater growth delays with amphetamine, while others describe equivalent deficits with amphetamine and methylphenidate formulations. Deficits occur across the dose range but are positively correlated with increasing medication doses. One study suggested that a medication holiday over one summer did not improve growth velocity, but holidays over two summers led to improved growth rates.[3] Weekend medication holidays do not appear to effect growth rates, but discontinuing medication over extended school breaks may have some benefit.

The main clinical issue is whether the potential for short-term decreases in expected growth outweigh the potential benefits of treating a child's ADHD. Given the known risks associated with the disorder, this assessment generally favors providing medication.

Can ADHD Medications Cause Sudden Death?

Intermittent reports of sudden death in patients taking ADHD medications contribute to ongoing concerns about potential cardiac risks. In response to reports of sudden death in patients taking mixed amphetamine salts, officials in Canada removed the drug from their market, although this was subsequently reversed. Stimulants are associated with increases of 2–5 mm Hg systolic and 1–3 mm Hg diastolic blood pressures, as well as small but significant increases in average pulse rate. These increases might be expected to create increased risk for cardiovascular problems. However, after considerable study, there is general consensus that the frequency of sudden cardiac death in young patients treated with ADHD medications is within the expected rate for the general population.[4]

Clinical medication trials are too small and short in duration to assess long-term cardiac risks. However, several large epidemiological studies provide reassurance. In one study of over 170,000 youth, there were no differences in rates of cardiovascular events such as myocardial infarctions, cerebrovascular accidents, or sudden cardiac death in individuals prescribed ADHD medication lacking known cardiac risk factors.[5] There were no differences between those prescribed or not prescribed stimulants or in those taking methylphenidate versus amphetamine. A second study of more than 440,000 young and middle-aged adults also failed to demonstrate any differences in cardiac risks associated with current, remote, or no stimulant use.[6]

Frequent reports of sudden cardiac death in athletes and other young and apparently healthy individuals are also attributable to general population risk. Cardiac risk screening is a major reason for physical examinations prior to participation in competitive sports (see Chapter 6). Viewed in these terms, cardiac risks associated with ADHD medications are comparable to those engendered by youth recreational sports and other common physical activities.

The US Food and Drug Administration warns that "sudden death has been reported in association with CNS stimulant treatment at usual doses in children and adolescents with structural cardiac abnormalities or other serious heart problems." Current practice standards require assessment prior to initiation of ADHD medications of any personal history of syncope, dizziness, palpitations, or chest pain, any family history early sudden cardiac death, and completion of a careful cardiac examination (see Chapter 6). The FDA also recommends intermittent clinical pulse and blood pressure monitoring in patients prescribed ADHD medications (see Chapter 10).

Should an Electrocardiogram Be Obtained Before Starting Medication?

Some clinicians routinely obtain electrocardiograms (EKGs) prior to initiating medication, and American Heart Association guidelines support this when clinically indicated. However, no compelling data suggest that routine EKGs effectively screen for early sudden cardiac death, and the American Academy of Pediatrics does not endorse routine screening prior to initiation of ADHD medication.[7] Rather than obtaining an EKG, it is preferable to screen patients based on history and cardiac examination findings and refer individuals deemed at risk for more comprehensive assessment by an appropriate specialist (see Chapter 6).

Can ADHD Medications Cause Birth Defects?

With increasing ADHD pharmacotherapy in older adolescents and adults, concerns have emerged about potential medication risks to a developing fetus or young infant. Women are generally advised to avoid or minimize medication use while pregnant or breastfeeding. At times, however, the mother's clinical needs warrant ongoing treatment. Concerns also exist about women who are attempting to become pregnant or are unaware of an early pregnancy.

Most clinical trials exclude pregnant participants, and no studies have examined potential teratogenic effects of ADHD medications. Animal studies suggest that stimulants cross the placenta and enter fetal circulation, although direct human data are unavailable. No teratogenic effects were seen in rats, but an increased incidence of spina bifida occurred in rabbits with methylphenidate exposure 40 times the usual therapeutic doses.

One report identified 180 women who had taken methylphenidate during their first trimester of pregnancy.[8] Of these, four children with major birth defects were observed, a rate within the expected population range.

Although limited, these data provide reassurance regarding stimulant-related birth defect risks.

The solubility and low molecular weight of methylphenidate suggests that it enters breast milk, but drug amounts available for infant ingestion vary with maternal dose, absorption, and metabolism. Estimates of relative infant dose, defined as the ratio of the amount ingested by baby and mother, are within a range generally accepted as safe.

Available evidence suggests that there is no to very little risk of fetal drug exposure in the earliest weeks of gestation, so there is no apparent need to stop medication in anticipation of pregnancy.[8] A decision to continue or not during pregnancy or breastfeeding must balance individual clinical necessity and potential risk.

Can ADHD Medications Cause Cancer?

One small study in 12 children found an association with methylphenidate and chromosomal abnormalities in peripheral lymphocytes.[9] This raised concern over possible increased cancer risk with methylphenidate treatment. Children served as their own controls, with assessments of chromosome damage performed before and after medication use. Several follow-up studies using similar methods failed to detect chromosomal change.

Another investigation of over 20,000 individuals with ADHD evaluated drug use profiles and emergent cancer rates.[10] Medications examined included methylphenidate, amphetamine, other ADHD medications, antidepressants, antipsychotics, and combination therapies. No increased risk for cancer was detected for methylphenidate, any other drug, or any drug class.

Larger studies and longer periods of observation would be useful in evaluating potential links between ADHD medications and cancer risk, but current evidence does not support any association.

Do ADHD Medications Lead to Drug Abuse and Addiction?

News media frequently report widespread abuse of ADHD medications. While these stories raise legitimate concerns, they conflate problems related to stimulants prescribed for ADHD and other stimulants, such as Ecstasy, cocaine, and "street" methamphetamine, and fail to distinguish patterns of use, including abuse, misuse, and diversion. Drug "use" includes taking medication as prescribed to reduce ADHD symptoms, for recreational mind-altering effects such as intoxication or euphoria, for other purposes such as weight loss, or for performance enhancement. Strictly defined, "abuse" refers to a pattern of use consistent with the *DSM-5* definition of substance use disorder, which requires use in situations that create risk for harm, failure to meet personal obligations, or symptoms of tolerance, withdrawal, or dependence. "Diversion" is the transfer of medication to someone for whom it is not prescribed. "Misuse" is the taking of medication by someone for whom it is not prescribed or in ways not prescribed.

Rates of misuse and diversion are estimated at 4.5% of middle and high school students. Numerous studies suggest that between 2% and 16% of college student misuse ADHD medications.[11] Of students with ADHD, 25% to 30% describe being asked to sell their medication and 11% has done so. The majority of misuse among college-age youth is for purposes of academic performance enhancement. About 30% is for recreational purposes, that is, to get high. Medications are most commonly obtained from peers or family members, and their highest use is during exam periods or other times of high academic stress. In one study, a third of students misusing ADHD medication stole it, 20% faked ADHD symptoms to obtain it from a physician, and 5% bought it from an Internet pharmacy.

Misuse is more common at colleges in the Northeast and those with highly competitive admissions. Misuse occurs more frequently among students who are White, male, in fraternities, and have lower grades. Students involved in misuse and diversion of ADHD medications have higher rates of alcohol, tobacco, and recreational drug use, and other difficulties with substance use disorders and conduct-disordered behavior. Even when misused, most medications are taken orally. Medications are also commonly crushed and either injected or taken intranasally by those seeking intoxication.

Physicians prescribing ADHD medications should be mindful of patient groups at highest risk for diversion and misuse. Physicians should counsel high-risk patients about the need to safeguard prescriptions and obtain commitments that medication will not be diverted or shared. Extended-release and pro-drug formulations have less risk for abuse than immediate-release stimulants and are preferred options when the potential for misuse is a clinical concern. Physicians can also choose nonstimulant ADHD treatments when the risks for abuse and misuse exceed what can be managed with confidence.

Related issues are whether patients become addicted to their ADHD medications and if stimulant treatment creates future risk for other substance use. Longitudinal studies clearly show there is no risk of stimulant addiction or increased risk for substance use disorders in young adult previously treated for ADHD.[12] Other evidence suggests that stimulant treatment in childhood and adolescence protects against the increased risk of substance use that occurs in untreated ADHD (see Chapters 3 and 11), although these results are less clear.[13] No data support withholding ADHD medications for fear of causing substance use difficulties.

Do People Fake ADHD to Get Drugs?

Many clinicians, particularly those who do not assess and treat childhood ADHD, remain suspicious that adults requesting evaluations are feigning symptoms to obtain medication or other special services. Consistent with this, one study suggests that half of university students presenting for ADHD assessments exaggerate symptoms.[11] Consequently, many university health services refuse to evaluate students for ADHD and many practitioners refuse to prescribe ADHD medication for adults.

Several approaches are proposed to differentiate adults with true ADHD from those who are feigning symptoms to pursue various benefits.[11] Solicitation of clinical information from multiple sources, including parents, employers, spouses, partners, and friends, as well as review past school and medical records, is a critical step in confirming a diagnosis. Consistent use of self and other-informant rating scales, neuropsychological assessments, computerized tests of attention such as the Conners' Continuous Performance Test (CPT), and quantitative electroencephalography (EEG) have been proposed, but none of these has been effective in improving diagnostic accuracy. Additional research and development of validated biological markers are sorely needed. Presently, the clinician must rely on individual judgment to assess the potential benefits and risks of prescribing treatment in any given patient.

Should ADHD Medications Be Prescribed If Someone Is Using Recreational Drugs or Alcohol?

Recreational drug use is common among individuals with ADHD. Clinicians must decide whether to provide prescription medication to patients who are currently abusing other psychoactive substances. In addition to heightened concerns about misuse and illicit diversion, there is a potential for negative drug interactions and worsening of underlying problems with concomitant prescription and illicit substance use. Conversely, in some appropriate treatment could potentially improve substance use.

There are no clear consensus guidelines for prescribing ADHD medications with concurrent psychoactive substance use or use disorders.[14] Most ADHD clinical trials exclude participants with significant active use, so empirical evidence to direct treatment is lacking. A decision to treat or not depends on several factors, including the degree of diagnostic uncertainty, potential overlap of ADHD and substance use symptoms, risk of substance use exacerbation, and the clinician's ability to monitor prescription compliance and response. The type of drugs used, patterns, frequency and consequences of use, and degree of dependence are all factors to be considered on a case-by-case basis.

Available research is both reassuring and disappointing. Treatment of ADHD during concurrent recreational drug use does not appear to worsen any substance use disorder.[15] Both stimulants and atomoxetine are proven effective in multiple studies for reducing ADHD symptoms even during active recreational drug use. However, ADHD treatment does not appear to improve substance use itself.[15]

Delaying ADHD treatment until after substance use issues are resolved facilitates more accurate ADHD diagnosis and assessment of treatment outcomes without confounding effects of other psychoactive drugs. However, given that some degree of recreational substance use is normative, strict insistence on a sobriety prior to diagnosis and initiation of treatment is likely to be counterproductive. Conversely, very frequent and heavy recreational use of psychoactive substances is apt to obscure any potential ADHD treatment benefit. If the clinician determines that treatment is appropriate, proper documentation of target symptoms, prescription information, and treatment outcomes in the medical record is essential to good practice.

Is It Useful to Get Stimulant Blood Levels?

Some clinicians obtain laboratory measurement of stimulant plasma levels as part of clinical management. Although these tests are readily available from commercial laboratories, no standard therapeutic window for medication response has been established and no relationship between plasma concentration and behavioral or cardiovascular response has been demonstrated. Laboratory assessment can document medication compliance on a given day, but it does not provide any additional value in routine clinical care.

Do Medications Stop Working?

Separate from questions about acute tolerance to stimulants over the course of daily treatment is the larger issue of potential loss of medication benefit with long-term use. Parents and patients often inquire about the risk of dependency or addiction to ADHD medications. Despite US FDA warnings that long-term use of stimulants can lead to dependence, longitudinal studies convincingly demonstrate that patients prescribed ADHD medications do not become addicted to them.[12] Whether or not some patients develop long-term medication tolerance is a more nuanced question for which available evidence fails to provide a clear answer.

In numerous open-label stimulant studies of 1–2 years duration, most participants do not require medication adjustments once optimal doses are established. Similarly, many patients are treated clinically for many years without any need for dose or medication changes, suggesting that long-term medication tolerance does not occur. This contrasts with evidence from the MTA Study in which participants in the optimal medication management arm typically required ongoing dose adjustments to maximize benefits.[16] It was unclear whether this reflected the need for increasing doses as patients grew or the possibility of long-term tolerance effects. While not common, some patients treated clinically do complain that previously effective medications stop working. It is also possible that some patients discontinue therapy due to lack of sustained effects. Finally, the phenomenon of "rebound hyperactivity" in which patients exhibit symptoms at or worse than baseline during late afternoon when medications are losing effect is well described, and it further suggests that stimulants cause acute brain changes that might negatively affect behavior.

Although development of long-term tolerance does not seem to be a major clinical concern, it might be in some cases. One small study provided a potential physiological explanation for tolerance effects. Investigators using positron emission tomography (PET) and a dopamine transporter ligand assessed the effects of 12 months of methylphenidate treatment on striatal dopamine transporter densities.[17] Dopamine transporter densities increased in participants on stimulant therapy, suggesting that brain adaptations occur with treatment. Authors hypothesized that upregulation of the dopamine transporter system could lead to increased symptoms and decreased medication effects. The study did not assess dopamine signaling in the prefrontal cortex, nor did it address noradrenergic mechanisms. Furthermore, clinical implications of these changes have not been elucidated. The potential for long-term tolerance and brain changes resulting from stimulant use requires further investigation. Absent a clear understanding of this phenomenon, standard clinical approaches to medication adjustment remain the best course when treatments cease to provide positive effects.

References

1. Faraone SV, Biederman J, Morley CP, Spencer TJ. Effect of stimulants on height and weight: a review of the literature. *J Am Acad Child Adolesc Psychiatry.* 2008;47:994–1009.

2. Swanson JM, Elliott GR, Greenhill LL, et al. The effects of long-term stimulant medication on growth rates across 3 years in the MTA follow-up. *J Am Acad Child Adolesc Psychiatry.* 2007;46:1015–1027.

3. Kratochvil CJ, Wilens TR, Greenhill LL, et al. Effects of long-term atomoxetine treatment for young children with attention-deficit/hyperactivity disorder. *J Am Acad Child Adolesc Psychiatry.* 2006;45:919–927.

4. Hammerness P, Perrin JM, Shelley-Abrahamson R, Wilens TR. Cardiovascular risk of stimulant treatment in pediatric attention-deficit/hyperactivity disorder: update and clinical recommendations. *J Am Acad Child Adolesc Psychiatry.* 2011;50:978–990.

5. Olfson M, Huang C, Gerhard T, et al. Stimulants and cardiovascular events in youth with attention-deficit/hyperactivity disorder. *J Amer Acad Child Adolesc Psychiatry.* 2012;51:147–156.

6. Habel LA, Cooper WO, Sox CM, et al. ADHD medications and risk of serious cardiovascular events in young and middle-aged adults. *JAMA.* 2011;306:2673–2683.

7. Perrin JM, Friedman RA, Knilans TK, Black Box Working Group, Section on Cardiology and Cardiac Surgery. Cardiovascular monitoring and stimulant drugs for attention-deficit/hyperactivity disorder. *Pediatrics.* 2008;122:451–453.

8. Dideriksen D, Pottegard A, Hallas J, Aagaard L, Damkier P. First trimester *in utero* exposure to methylphenidate. *Basic Clin Pharmacol Tox.* 2012;112:73–76.

9. El-Zein RA, Abdel-Rahman SZ, Hay MJ, et al. Cytogenic effects in children treated with methylphenidate. *Cancer Lett.* 2005;230:284–291.

10. Steinhausen HC, Helenius D. The association between medication for attention deficit hyperactivity disorder and cancer. *J Child Adolesc Psychopharmacol.* 2013;23:208–213.

11. Rabiner DL. Stimulant prescription cautions: addressing misuse, diversion and malingering. *Curr Psychiatry Rep.* 2013;15:375.

12. Barkley RA, Fischer M, Smallish L, Fletcher K. Does the treatment of attention-deficit/hyperactivity disorder with stimulants contribute to drug use/abuse?: a 13-year prospective study. *Pediatrics.* 2003;111:97–109.

13. Wilens TE, Adamson J, Monuteaux MC, et al. Effect of prior stimulant treatment for attention-deficit/hyperactivity disorder on subsequent risk for

cigarette smoking and alcohol and drug use disorders in adolescents. *Arch Pediatr Adolesc Med.* 2008;162:916–921.

14. Upadhyaya HP. Managing attention-deficit/hyperactivity disorder in the presence of substance use disorder. *J Clin Psychiatry.* 2007;68:23–30.

15. Mariani JJ, Levin FR. Treatment strategies for co-occurring ADHD and substance use disorders. *Am J Addict.* 2007;16:45–54.

16. MTA Cooperative Group. National Institute of Mental Health Multimodal Treatment Study of ADHD follow-up: 24-month outcomes of treatment strategies for attention-deficit/hyperactivity disorder. *Pediatrics.* 2004;113:754–761.

17. Wang GJ, Volkow ND, Wigal T, et al. Long-term stimulant treatment affects brain dopamine transporter levels in patients with attention deficit hyperactivity disorder. *PloS One.* 2013;8:e63023.

Further Reading

Bolea-Alamanac BM, Green A, Verma G, Maxwell P, Davies SJ. Methylphenidate use in pregnancy and lactation: a systematic review of evidence. *Br J Clin Pharmacol.* 2014;77:96–101.

Cooper WO, Habel LA, Sox CM, et al. ADHD drugs and serious cardiovascular events in children and young adults. *N Eng J Med.* 2011;365:1896–1904.

Faraone SV, Wilens TE. Effect of stimulant medications for attention-deficit/hyperactivity disorder on later substance use and the potential for stimulant misuse, abuse, and diversion. *J Clin Psychiatry.* 2006;68:15–22.

Chapter 13

Complementary and Alternative Medicine Therapies

> ## Key Points
>
> - There is tremendous lay interest in complementary and alternative medicine approaches to ADHD.
> - The only complementary or alternative ADHD treatment with sufficient evidence to support its use is omega-3 fatty acid supplementation, which given a small positive effect size is recommended as a potentially useful adjunctive therapy with standard pharmacotherapy.
> - Patients and families who refuse established treatments in lieu of complementary and alternative approaches risk increased negative consequences of untreated ADHD.

There is tremendous interest in complementary and alternative medicine (CAM) treatments for ADHD. Parents and patients are often concerned about medication safety and prefer therapies that avoid pharmacotherapy or are viewed as "natural." Some patients respond poorly to medication. Even when beneficial, medications have side effects, rarely normalize behavior, and have little evidence of long-term benefit. By definition, complementary treatments are used in conjunction with standard therapies, while alternative treatments are used in place of them. CAM treatments might be reasonable options when patients fail or have inadequate responses to conventional therapies. It is estimated that over 60% of children and large numbers of adults have used CAM treatments for ADHD.[1]

Despite their popularity, almost all CAM therapies have failed to meet criteria as evidence-based treatments or demonstrated sufficient benefit to support recommendations for use (Box 13.1).[1,2] While there are many published studies of CAM treatments for ADHD, most are methodologically flawed. Sample sizes are small, randomization is suspect, control groups are absent or poorly designed, patients are inadequately diagnosed, and articles are written by investigators with financial incentives to promote treatments. Positive meta-analyses are commonly based on ratings by individuals with strong pre-existing beliefs in treatment efficacy or significant time investments in providing the intervention. These raters, usually parents or therapists, tend to inflate treatment effect sizes. Results are also commonly confounded by medication use. For almost all CAM treatments, positive effects vanish when based on blinded assessments in unmedicated participants.[2]

Box 13.1 Evidence for Complementary and Alternative ADHD Treatments Based on Blinded Ratings

Sufficient Evidence Supporting Recommendation for Use
Omega-3 fatty acid supplementation
Mean effect size = .16, suggesting possible role as adjunctive therapy

Lack Sufficient Evidence Supporting Recommendation for Use

Acupuncture	Massage therapy
Amino acid supplements	Mindfulness-based meditation, yoga
Caffeine	Nutraceutical supplements
Chiropractic therapy	Repetitive transcranial magnetic stimulation
Cognitive training	Restriction/elimination diets
Electroencephalographic neurofeedback	Sensory integration therapy
Exercise	Vision therapy
Homeopathy	Vitamin and mineral supplements
Interactive metronome therapy	

Source: Data taken from Sonuga-Barke et al.[2]

The primary risk of most CAM treatments is the failure to administer standard therapies with proven efficacy and safety. Families can devote substantial effort and resources pursuing nonmedication interventions that lack any evidence of positive benefit. Some CAM treatments themselves have risks for toxicity or other adverse outcomes. Clinicians should maintain awareness about CAM research so that they can properly advise patients on treatment choices.

Restriction/Elimination Diets

There is widespread belief that ADHD is caused by or can be treated with diet. Most research on dietary interventions has serious methodological flaws, including inadequate comparison groups, investigator and publication bias, unblinded or biased parent raters, and a lack of confirmation by blinded symptom reports. Of all restricted diets, only artificial food coloring elimination has shown significant benefit on blinded ratings. However, long-term adherence to restricted diets is extremely difficult, can lead to nutritional deficiencies, and appears justified only in small subsets of patients with particular sensitivities.[3]

Feingold Diet

Beginning in the 1970s, some proposed that childhood hyperactivity was caused by increased sensitivity to certain foods. Dr. Ben Feingold, a pediatrician and allergist, wrote several books espousing dietary treatment for childhood behavioral problems that eliminated synthetic food colors, flavors, and preservatives, and foods containing salicylates, such as certain nuts and fruits. Although Feingold originally reported behavioral improvements in over 50% of treated children, subsequent research revealed that many foods in his diet actually contained salicylates. Numerous blinded controlled trials failed to show any benefits, with the exception of a small group of preschool-age youth who reacted negatively when additives and preservatives were added blindly to their diets. Although proponents continue to debate these largely negative conclusions, there is no current evidence suggesting the Feingold Diet is effective for ADHD.[1]

Oligoantigenic Elimination Diet

Other diet strategies propose that hyperactivity is an abnormal reaction to an array of certain foods, including cow's milk, cheese, eggs, nuts, wheat products, and citrus. One highly publicized approach touts an "oligoantigenic" diet comprised of a very limited number of supposedly hypoallergenic foods such as lamb, chicken, certain vegetables, salt, pepper, and particular food supplements. Although meta-analysis suggests that 30% of children would benefit from oligoantigenic elimination, studies themselves have major limitations.[4] Treatments required extensive involvement from unblinded parents. Control conditions were poorly designed. Concomitant medications were not controlled. Positive effects disappeared when restricted to blinded ratings. Practically, this diet is too restrictive for long-term maintenance and carries substantial risk for nutritional deficiencies.[1]

Sugar-Restricted Diets

There are persistent beliefs that eating refined sugar causes hyperactivity. However, numerous blinded studies failed to detect any behavioral effects from dietary sugar.[1] In blinded comparisons of sugar versus placebo, mothers report increased motor activity when they believed their children ate sugar regardless of what was actually eaten.[5] Diets high in refined sugar are clearly related to obesity and other health risks. As a matter of good health maintenance, clinicians should advise parents and patients to maintain diets containing wide varieties of lightly processed foods. However, nothing suggests that occasional consumption of refined sugar or other treats is associated with meaningful health risks. No evidence suggests that restriction of dietary sugar improves ADHD.

Artificial Food Coloring

Artificial food coloring elimination is the one restricted diet with some level of scientifically meaningful support. Positive effects are demonstrated on blinded and unblinded ratings, although these lose significance in meta-analyses restricted to studies with low or no medication use.[2] Benefits might be strongest in groups selected for food sensitivities, which some suggest is related to individual genetic risk. Regulatory authorities in the United Kingdom required restrictive labeling for artificial food colorings following reports of diet-related behavioral improvements in preschool children. The US Food and Drug Administration (FDA) found insufficient scientific data to warrant this approach.

One meta-analysis concluded that up to 8% of ADHD symptoms in the general population might be attributed to artificial food coloring.[4] Food coloring restrictions yield small treatment effects, much smaller than ADHD medications. Even these small effects might be overestimates given the strong likelihood of publication bias against negative reports. There is no consensus on which additives putatively cause risk, although yellow dye 5 containing tartrazine has garnered much attention. Artificial food colorings have no nutritional value. While any benefit from their restriction is likely to be small, there are no apparent harms if parents choose to avoid them.

Dietary Supplements

Essential Fatty Acids

Essential fatty acid (EFA) supplementation is another one of a few CAM therapies with proven benefit.[6] Over a dozen trials have been conducted, with wide variations in design, comparison controls, and dose. Some of the largest only assessed ADHD symptoms and had no systematic approach for assigning an actual ADHD diagnosis. Study dropout rates are high, and there are concerns about the fishy taste of supplements, which can lead to treatment unblinding. Meta-analysis suggests mean effect sizes in the range of .16, which are small but remain significant for both unblinded and blinded ratings and when studies allowing concomitant stimulants were eliminated.[2] A trial of EFA supplementation might be justified if a parent strongly opposes stimulants. However, given that treatment effect sizes are small, evidence suggests that EFA supplements, if used, be given adjunctively with conventional ADHD medication.

Main dietary sources of EFA include cold-water fish, walnuts, almonds, dark green leafy vegetables, whole grain foods, eggs, and olive oil. Two main types are omega-3 fatty acids, which include docosahexanoic acid (DHA) and eicosapentaenoic acid (EPA), and omega-6 fatty acids, which include arachidonic acid and γ-linolenic acid (GLA). Supplements vary widely in their rations of omega-3 and omega-6 compounds. Optimal formulations appear to contain more omega-3 EFAs, particulalry EPA. Optimal doses are in the range of 1,000 mg of omega-3 daily. Primary benfits appear to be on improved attention and behavior, and require 3 to 4 months of consistent therapy. EFA supplementation has other presumed benefits, particulalry on cardiovascular health, and is presumed to be safe when avoiding preparations that contain mercury.[3]

Vitamin and Mineral Supplements

While a general recommendation for multivitamin use is supported for all children with dietary deficiencies, there is no evidence to suggest that vitamin therapy is useful for ADHD.[3] Children who took a daily multivitamin at standard doses meeting minimal daily requirements had improved nonverbal intelligence, concentration, and motor control. However, these benefits were seen primarily in children with poor diets and were not specific to ADHD. Some children with ADHD typically have poor dietary habits that could benefit with multivitamin supplementation.

Claims for ADHD benefits are also made for various individual vitamins and minerals, both with standard- and mega-dose therapy. None of these claims has been studied systematically. Positive results from open trials from zinc were not confirmed in blinded studies. Iron supplementation has been useful only in children with iron deficiencies. Iron-related improvements in children without anemia were noted only on parent, but not teacher ratings. Given the toxicities that are associated with high doses of iron, magnesium, and other minerals, as well as high-dosed vitamin therapy, supplementation should be limited to those with documented insufficiencies.[7]

Amino Acids

Several short-term studies of various amino acids as potential ADHD treatments have been conducted.[1] The most commonly studied agent is acetyl L-carnitine (ALC), an amino acid derivative. Other amino acids tested include gamma-aminobutyric acid (GABA), glycine, L-tyrosine, taurine, L-tyrosine, 5-hydroxytryptophan (5-HTP), dimethylaminoethanol (DMAE), and s-adenosyl-L-methionine (SAMe). None have demonstrated improved ADHD and none are recommended as ADHD therapy.

Other Supplements

Nutraceuticals are products derived from food, including herbs, isolated nutrients, dietary supplements, and other sources, which are taken in medicinal forms not associated with food and are presumed to have physiological or health benefits. In addition to supplements previously described, numerous others are marketed for improving attention, overactivity, or ADHD. These products are very popular among parents and patients who wish to avoid prescription drugs and use treatments they believe are "natural."

Various nutraceuticals are marketed individually or as components of proprietary blends. Few have any proven benefit and some are associated with potential risks.[1] Herbal supplements are derived from flowers or other plant products. Extracts of Gingko biloba are mild monoamine oxidase and catecholamine reuptake inhibitors. There are some benefits of Gingko for dementia, but ADHD effects are uncertain. St. John's Wort, another popular nutraceutical, is used for a variety of reasons, but it has no demonstrated ADHD benefit. Pycnogenol, derived from pine tree bark, reportedly increases blood circulation, but it is ineffective for ADHD. Glyconutrients are plant-based carbohydrates, which reportedly support brain cell function and connectivity, but ADHD studies have significant methodological difficulties and unclear results. Valerian and kava-kava exhibit gabaminergic activity with associated calming effects, but it has no demonstrated utility for ADHD. Kava use has been implicated with risk for liver toxicity. Melatonin has some value as a sleep aid, but it has no proven ADHD benefit. Several proprietary blends, including FOCUSFactor®, AttentiveChild™, On Task™, and Kids Calm Multi, are marketed as treatments for behavioral problems and hyperactivity but have no scientific evidence supporting this use.

The FDA does not regulate nutraceuticals and other supplements in the same way as prescription medications. There is no requirement for makers of these products to demonstrate efficacy and safety data in support of their health-promoting claims. There are no guarantees about product quality control and some products contain components that are not described in their labels.

Caffeine

Many believe that caffeine is beneficial for ADHD. The stimulating effects of caffeine rely on very different mechanisms of action than ADHD medications. Caffeine can lead to wakefulness and brief increases in attention, but it does not have any more than negligible effects on ADHD symptoms.[8]

Homeopathy

Homeopathic approaches to disease have been employed for over 150 years. In homeopathy, very small quantities of substances that cause particular symptoms in healthy individuals are given to patients with the expectation that those symptoms will be reduced. Systematic reviews of homeopathic research, including several trials in ADHD, have failed to demonstrate any benefits.[9]

Neuropsychological Treatments

Cognitive Training

Cognitive training approaches to ADHD attempt to strengthen neuropsychological processes seen as deficient in the disorder, such as attention or working memory. Several commercially available, computer-based, proprietary programs are designed to improve cognitive functioning and, by extension, ADHD. One of the most popular is CogMed, which provides training in either verbal or spatial working memory. Other programs purport to provide attention training, cognitive remediation, executive function training, and enhanced cognitive control.

A course of CogMed requires 25 sessions of 30–45 minutes each, usually over 5 weeks. Numerous studies report benefits from CogMed as well as other cognitive training therapies. Positive outcomes are reported for unblinded parent and teacher reports, but these effects disappear with blinded ratings.[2] In several reports, CogMed has been associated with improved working memory performance on computerized tests, but these results do not correlate with improved ADHD symptoms. The current evidence base does not support use of CogMed or other cognitive training programs as ADHD treatments.

Electroencephalographic Neurofeedback/Biofeedback

For over 20 years, EEG neurofeedback has been one of the most popular CAM treatments for ADHD. Neurofeedback training is based on observations that some individuals with ADHD exhibit increased theta and decreased beta spectral power during electroencephalography (EEG). Increased theta activity is associated with inattention, impulsivity, and hyperactivity, while decreased beta activity is associated with poor concentration and underarousal. Methylphenidate increases beta activity in medication responders, but not in nonresponders. During neurofeedback training, patients undergo EEG monitoring, usually via scalp electrodes, and receive real-time visual feedback, typically on a computer screen, about patterns of brain activity. By responding to this feedback, patients self-regulate to decrease theta and increase beta wave activity. Treatments occur in 30- to 60-minute sessions conducted two to three times weekly over a course of approximately 13 weeks.

There are over a dozen double-blind controlled studies of EEG neurofeedback for ADHD. One meta-analysis reported moderate treatment effects comparable to results found typically with nonstimulant ADHD medications.[10] However, studies included in the analysis suffered numerous limitations. Treatments were not standardized. Many lacked true "triple-blinding" of children, parents, and therapists to treatment assignment, leading to inadequate blinding of "sham" control treatments. Concomitant medication received inconsistent consideration. While ratings from parents, who were generally unblinded and highly invested in treatment success, demonstrated statistically significant improvements, these findings were not replicated by blinded teacher reports.[2] One well-designed, well-controlled, triple-blinded sham-comparison study funded by the National Institute of Mental Health failed to show any difference between active treatment and control groups.[11] EEG neurofeedback is an expensive, time-intensive therapy that remains unproven for ADHD. Despite its widespread popularity, neither the American Academy of Pediatrics nor the American Academy of Child and Adolescent Psychiatry endorses its use.

Mind-Body Therapies

Acupuncture

Acupuncture is reasonably safe and increasingly used outside of Asian cultures for a range of indications. Use of acupuncture for ADHD is based on Chinese beliefs that the disorder arises from physical imbalances that are corrected by treatment. Scientific studies of acupuncture treatment do not support its use in ADHD.[12]

Chiropractic Adjustment

There is inherent appeal for chiropractic adjustment as an ADHD treatment, particularly for those who oppose or are reluctant to use pharmacotherapy. Publications about chiropractic interventions for ADHD are limited in number and are mostly case reports that suffer significant design flaws, including small sample sizes, inadequate diagnostic assessment, and inadequate control groups. The purported mechanism of action, that is, restoration of dysfunctional brain systems through correcting subluxations of the spinal column, is not consistent with known ADHD pathophysiology. There is no scientific evidence supporting chiropractic interventions for ADHD.[1]

Exercise

It is reasonable to assume that exercise and increased physical activity would benefit individuals who suffer from motoric overactivity and restlessness. Numerous studies suggest that regular exercise has positive effects on behavior, cognition, and mood. Only a small subset, however, have examined a specific role for exercise in ADHD, and these suffer from small sample sizes and inadequate control comparisons. While broad recommendations for increased physical activity might facilitate general overall health, there are insufficient data to support exercise as a general ADHD treatment.

Interactive Metronome Training

Interactive metronome training was introduced by occupational therapists as an ADHD treatment in the early 1990s. The intervention requires patients to match the rhythmic beat of computer-generated tones by tapping their feet or clapping their hands and is purported to improve attention, concentration, and physical coordination. Published research findings are scant and limited by small sample sizes, inadequate control groups, and investigator bias. The evidence base is inadequate to support its use as an ADHD therapy.[1]

Meditation, Mindfulness, Yoga, and Massage

Although there is widespread interest, very few studies have examined medi-tation, mindfulness training, yoga, or massage therapy for ADHD. Published reports utilize small adult samples and lack adequate controls. There are gen-erally two types of meditation studies, mantra meditation and yoga. No dif-ferences have been found between groups assigned to meditation or usual medication treatment, although sample sizes in these studies lack sufficient power to detect differences that might be really present.[13] These studies should not be misconstrued to imply that meditation and medication effects are equal. One adult study of mindfulness training had loose entry criteria and claimed to show positive change on cognitive testing, but it was uncontrolled. Authors of these studies convey strong convictions that the interventions are effective. However, there is insufficient evidence from objective reviews to claim positive effects for ADHD or to support recommendations as ADHD treatments.

Repetitive Transcranial Magnetic Stimulation

Repetitive transcranial magnetic stimulation (rTMS) utilizes an electromagnet to generate a low-grade electrical current across the scalp, which is believed to stimulate small areas of the brain leading to increased brain signaling. Some positive results with rTMS are evidenced in treatment-refractory depression and patients recovering from stroke. Studies in ADHD are limited to small adult samples and fail to provide sufficient evidence to support rTMS as an ADHD treatment.[1]

Sensory Integration Training

"Sensory processing disorder" is a term used by occupational therapists for individuals who are overly sensitive to a range of environmental stimuli, including some with ADHD. The term is not a recognized medical disorder. Sensory integration training comprises physical exercises that are intended to improve the body's sense of its relationship to external space. As with studies of interactive metronome treatment, published reports suffer from significant methodological flaws, particularly overly broad inclusion criteria, small sample sizes, inadequate controls, and investigator bias. There is no objective evidence base supporting sensory integration training for ADHD.[1]

Vision Therapy

Some behavioral optometrists offer vision therapy for a range of disorders that includes autism spectrum disorder, learning disorders, and ADHD. Exercises are practiced in the office and at home with the goal of training the eyes to remain focused on various visual stimuli. There is debate among optometrists as to whether vision therapy is effective for ADHD itself or undetected vision problems that frequently lead to misdiagnosis of ADHD. One double-blind sham-controlled study found support for treating convergence insufficiency, but no studies support its use in psychiatric disorders.[14] Neither the American Academy of Pediatrics or the Academy of Child and Adolescent Psychiatry recommends vision therapy in its ADHD practice guidelines.

References

1. Bader A, Adesman A. Complementary and alternative therapies for children and adolescents with ADHD. *Curr Op Pediatrics*. 2012;24:760–769.

2. Sonuga-Barke EJ, Brandeis D, Daley D, et al. Nonpharmacological interventions for ADHD: systematic review and meta-analysis of randomized controlled trials of dietary and psychological treatments. *Am J Psychiatry*. 2013;170:275–289.

3. Hurt EA, Arnold LE, Lofthouse N. Dietary and nutritional treatment for attention-deficit/hyperactivity disorder; current research support and recommendations for practitioners. *Curr Psychiatry Rep*. 2011;13:323–332.

4. Nigg JT, Lewis K, Edinger T, Falk M. Meta-analysis of attention-deficit/hyperactivity disorder or attention-deficit/hyperactivity disorder symptoms, restriction diet, and synthetic food color additives. *J Am Acad Child Adolesc Psychiatry*. 2012;51:86–97.

5. Hoover DW, Milich R. Effects of sugar ingestion expectancies on mother-child interactions. *J Abnorm Child Psychol*. 1994;22:501–515.

6. Bloch MH, Qawasmi A. Omega-3 fatty acid supplementation for the treatment of children with attention-deficit/hyperactivity disorder symptomatology: systematic review and meta-analysis. *J Am Acad Child Adolesc Psychiatry*. 2011;50:969–971.

7. Millichap JG, Yee MM. The diet factor in attention-deficit/hyperactivity disorder. *Pediatrics*. 2012;129:330–337.

8. Leon MR. Effects of caffeine on cognitive, psychomotor, and affective performance of children with attention-deficit/hyperactivity disorder. *J Atten Disord*. 2000;4:27–47.

9. Ernst E. Homeopathy: what does the "best" evidence tell us? *Med J Aust*. 2010;192:458–460.

10. Lofthouse N, Arnold LE, Hersch S, Hurt E, DeBeus A. A review of neurofeedback treatment for pediatric ADHD. *J Atten Disord*. 2012;16:351–372.

11. Arnold LE, Lofthouse N, Hersch S, et al. EEG neurofeedback for ADHD: double-blind sham-controlled pilot feasibility trial. *J Atten Disord*. 2013;17:410–419.

12. Li S, Yu B, Zhou D, et al. Acupuncture for attention deficit hyperactivity disorder (ADHD) in children and adolescents (review). *Cochrane Database Syst Rev*. 2011;4;CD007839.

13. Krisanaprakornkit T, Ngamjarus C, Witoonch C, Piyavhatkul N. Meditation therapies for attention deficit hyperactivity disorder (ADHD) (Review). *Cochrane Database Syst Rev.* 2010;6:CD006507.
14. Barnhardt C, Cotter SA, Mitchell GL, Scheiman M, Kulp MT, CITT Study Group. Symptoms in children with convergence insufficiency: before and after treatment. *Optom Vis Sci.* 2012;89:1512–1520.

Further Reading

Skokauskas N, McNicholas F, Masaud T, Frodl T. Complementary medicine for children and young people who have attention deficit hyperactivity disorder. *Curr Opin Psychiatry.* 2011;24:291–300.

Index

Page numbers followed by *f* or *t* indicate figures and tables.

CPSIA information can be obtained
at www.ICGtesting.com
Printed in the USA
BVHW03s0452180418
513670BV00006B/132/P

9 780199 969906